PLANNING AND ANALYSIS OF CLINICAL STUDIES

PLANNING AND ANALYSIS OF CLINICAL STUDIES

By

WALTER J. BURDETTE, Ph.D., M.D.

and

EDMUND A. GEHAN, Ph.D.

*The University of Texas M. D. Anderson Hospital and
Tumor Institute at Houston*

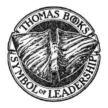

CHARLES C THOMAS · PUBLISHER
Springfield · Illinois · U.S.A.

Published and Distributed Throughout the World by
CHARLES C THOMAS • PUBLISHER
BANNERSTONE HOUSE
301-327 East Lawrence Avenue, Springfield, Illinois, U.S.A.
NATCHEZ PLANTATION HOUSE
735 North Atlantic Boulevard, Fort Lauderdale, Florida, U.S.A.

With THOMAS BOOKS *careful attention is given to all details of*
manufacturing and design. It is the Publisher's desire to present books
that are satisfactory as to their physical qualities and artistic possibilities
and appropriate for their particular use. THOMAS BOOKS will be true
to those laws of quality that assure a good name and good will.

PREFACE

THE CLINICIAN MUST CONTINUALLY EVALUATE DATA reported by others and the results of his own work in order to decide the most effective therapy for his patients. As an investigator, he must plan clinical and laboratory studies in such a way as to provide meaningful results with an economy of clinical resources. This implies a good understanding of the general principles of design and analysis. Intuitive conclusions, although valuable, must be supplemented not only by tests of significance but also by an understanding of clinical trials, appropriate size of sample, procedures for randomization, and some general knowledge of the design of experiments.

It is obvious that a single, short treatise cannot encompass the entire scope of statistics. However, it is possible to record most of what is ordinarily needed by the clinician when he designs and evaluates his own work and reviews that of others. This material is presented as an account of both retrospective and prospective studies in narrative style with appropriate examples. It should be acceptable to any practitioner of the clinical art, since the formulae and calculations are kept to a minimum. For those who wish to carry out their own calculations, requisite formulae and illustrative applications are presented in appendices with as much economy of words as seems consistent with clarity. A glossary of statistical terms and tables and graphs of *chi-square* and *t* are also included in this section.

It is hoped that this small volume will serve as a durable handbook, first, as a concise presentation of the contemporary approach to planning and evaluation of clinical investigations, and second, as a source of formulae, tables, and methods used most frequently in the actual analysis of data. The physician, investigator, graduate fellow, or medical student who reads it will recognize that his ingenuity and intuition are called upon as much as the application of significance tests in making a judgment about the best therapy available.

ACKNOWLEDGMENTS

THE AUTHORS are indebted to Professors William G. Cochran, Gertrude Cox, and George W. Snedecor and their publishers for permission to reproduce tables 9 and 33 from *Experimental Designs* (John Wiley and Sons)[13] and table 10 from *Statistical Methods* (Iowa State University Press)[46] respectively, and to Doctor James F. Crow[17] and the editors of the *Journal of the American Statistical Association* for the privilege of redrawing the chart of χ^2 and t. Gratitude is also expressed to the literary executor of the late Sir Ronald A. Fisher and to Oliver S. Boyd, Ltd., Edinburgh, for their permission to reprint tables of χ^2 and t from *Statistical Methods for Research Workers*.[22]

CONTENTS

TABLES

PLANNING AND ANALYSIS
OF CLINICAL STUDIES

I

INTRODUCTION

PRIOR TO THIS CENTURY, a scientific approach was not taken to the study of new medical treatments for several reasons, although comparative clinical studies were performed sporadically by accident or occasionally in a systematic way.[10] There was a special relationship between doctor and patient often (not) conducive to objective experimentation; lack of effective remedies made comparative studies unattractive; usually there was pronounced reverence for authority; and the obvious success of certain treatments such as reduction of dislocations and fractures made experimentation appear superfluous. In the thirteenth century, these complexities separating medicine from other scientific disciplines were recognized by Roger Bacon who suggested that "It is exceedingly difficult and dangerous to perform operations on the human body, wherefore it is more difficult to work in that science than any other . . . the operative and practical sciences which do their work on insensate bodies can multiply their experiments till they get rid of deficiency and errors, but a physician cannot do this because of the nobility of the material in which he works; for that body demands that no error be made in operating upon it and so experience (the experimental method) is difficult in medicine. Wherefore, physicians are to be excused for their defects more than are workers in the sciences."

The fortuitous clinical trial forced upon Paré[10, 40] by the lack of hot oil during the battle for the castle of Villaine is well known to surgeons. "I found those to whom I had applied the digestive medicament feeling but little pain, their wounds neither swollen nor inflamed, and having slept through the night. The others to whom I had applied the boiling oil were feverish with much pain and swelling about their wounds. Then I determined never again to burn thus so cruelly the poor wounded by arquebuses." Although the truth was grasped occasionally in flashes of recognition, such as this one, methods for assessing therapy were obviously not evident to practitioners. For example, Paré himself was guilty of condoning a test for supposed therapeutic properties of a bezoar stone on a hapless convict who was given corrosive sublimate with the prompt demise of the "volunteer." (His alternative punishment would have been equally terminal.)

In Europe, the obvious antimalarial action of cinchona was not accepted by the established practitioners of medicine at first and fell for decades into the hands of quacks and mountebanks. Even the decisive clinical trial by James Lind in 1747 demonstrating the usefulness of citrus fruits in the management of scurvy must not have been entirely convincing to the investigator, since he continued to attribute therapeutic properties to other remedies as well. By the eighteenth century, accounts of a more orderly approach to medical investigation, such as those of John Hunter and those of Withering on establishing the appropriate dosage of digitalis, began to appear. There were many rediscoveries of information known to physicians centuries earlier, and conclusions often were not justified by the evidence; but by the end of the eighteenth century the work of Jenner set the stage for a modern approach to clinical trials. This evolved slowly during the nineteenth century.

Large-scale trials, such as those sponsored by the League of Nations on the control of malaria in the early part of the twentieth century and those sponsored later by the United States Veterans' Administration on the treatment of tuberculosis and by the National Cancer Institute on the efficacy of chemotherapy in the management of cancer, were obvious signs that physicians had assimilated the principles of experimental design and were beginning to apply them to comparative problems in preventive and clinical medicine.

At first, retrospective analysis was a fashionable accessory for the academic clinician. Later it became obvious to all that minor as well as major adjustments in therapy that may be beneficial can be assessed when appropriate analytical methods are applied to clinical practice. Within the past decade, arguments have even been proposed that a physician has a moral obligation to conduct clinical experiments in certain circumstances. Armitage[3] states that "Frequently . . . there will be no convincing evidence as to the relative merits of the rival treatments. It is then generally felt to be no more unethical to treat some patients by each method than to use one treatment throughout. It has, indeed, been argued that the doctor is under a moral obligation to use the treatments available in such a way that he acquires information about their relative merits as quickly and effectively as possible." A similar argument has been advanced by Anscombe[2] who states that "It is not sufficient that a physician should give the best treatment he knows about; he is responsible for his own knowledge. Anything he can do to help improve his knowledge, and that of other physicians, is as much his duty as the correct application of his knowledge in treating patients. . . . In the improvement of knowledge, some patients will be ill treated, but if knowledge is not improved, all patients will be ill treated."

In general, society has endorsed experimentation in man for the solution of medical problems. Ideally, such experimentation should consist of well-designed experiments as well as possibly effective treatment for the individual patient. In no circumstances should the best interests of the individual be usurped in the conduct of the study.

II

GENERAL CONSIDERATIONS

TYPES OF STUDIES

THE MAIN TYPES OF PLANNED INVESTIGATIONS are prospective studies, retrospective studies and surveys. It is important to distinguish the conclusions that can be drawn from such studies. In prospective studies such as the comparative clinical trial, the choice of treatment for each individual is made by the investigator, whereas in the retrospective study or planned survey the observer has no control at all over what makes a particular individual fall in one group rather than another. Cogent conclusions about the causal effects of treatment can be drawn in comparative clinical trials which are designed so that the only difference in the groups of patients is in the treatment they receive. In retrospective studies, interesting conclusions can be drawn but further evidence is needed before the causality of an association may be asserted. Criteria for causality usually include specificity, consistency, strength of association, coherence and temporal relationship which are discussed more in detail in a later section. In planned surveys, the usual aim is to estimate the proportions of individuals possessing certain characteristics. Such studies * are mainly descriptive in nature.

GENERAL PRINCIPLES OF DESIGN

In planning a clinical study, whether prospective or retrospective, certain general principles require consideration.[1] First, it is obvious that the choice of surgical procedure or factor to be investigated (e.g., the effect of the prior status of the patient on operative mortality) must be made. Second, the experimental design must be chosen, particularly the units to be tested. Should the surgical procedure be attempted in animals first? If a surgical procedure is to be tried on human patients first, should it be attempted in severely ill or relatively well patients first? Third, the observations to be made on the experimental units must be chosen. For example, in a study of patients who undergo a radical mastectomy, should the end-point for analysis be the length of time from operation to the first recur-

* Death rates, prevalence rates, or incidence rates of various diseases are estimated in studies of mortality and morbidity. It may be desirable in such studies to make adjustments for age, and a good discussion of such studies and techniques of adjustment is given by Lilienfeld, Pederson, and Dowd.[85]

[6]

General Considerations
simplicity

rence of the disease or should "response" be the proportion of patients surviving five years following operation or the length of survival following operation? A different type of trial could be set up depending on the definition of response or end-point for analysis. Survival time is a completely objective end-point but death may not be caused by the patient's disease, and, if survival is long, patients may receive many different treatments for complications of their disease. The proportion of patients having remission of their disease (or remission of given duration) is a short-term end-point; but remission may be difficult to define for a particular disease, and it may not have a close relationship to survival time. In the course of a study using patients with cancer, decrease in tumor size may occur but at the cost of severe toxicity to the patient. For a particular trial, various objective end-points should be considered for their meaningfulness and the type and length of trial implied before a final selection is made.

These considerations clearly will have an important bearing on the outcome of the study. The ingenuity of the research worker and his ability to look at a problem from a number of different viewpoints are important factors in determining whether or not the study will be fruitful. There are certain general requirements for any good study. These are the absence of systematic error, the determination of the precision of estimates arising from the study, the range of the validity of the conclusions, the calculation of the uncertainty of any conclusions drawn, and simplicity. Each of these will be discussed in turn.

The *absence of systematic error* means that, if the study were done using a very large number of units, it would almost surely give a correct estimate of a difference in outcome between treatments or the importance *source systematic error* of some factor in determining the outcome of operation. An example that may clarify the point is a paper by Brinkley and Haybittle [8] who report the survival rates for patients with breast cancer treated by simple mastectomy in combination with irradiation and those treated by radical mastectomy and irradiation. The five-year crude survival rate for stage-II patients was 42 per cent for patients treated by radical mastectomy and irradiation and 62 per cent for patients treated by simple mastectomy and irradiation. Unfortunately, the types of operation were not randomized among patients. Therefore, the authors reported that there was a likelihood that selective factors were involved and that somewhat less advanced cases received the simple mastectomy. They write: "There is no answer to this criticism of comparability of groups and such a defect is almost certain to exist in any retrospective survey." If there were a systematic difference in the types of patients who were candidates for the simple and radical mastectomy, then no matter how many patients received each type of operation, an incorrect estimate would be obtained of the difference in five-year survival rates. Matching cases will help to overcome problems of this type in retrospective studies; and the randomization of cases should overcome this problem in prospective studies.

Estimates of effects should be sufficiently precise so that cogent conclusions can be drawn. When there is no systematic error in the study, an estimate such as the percentage of patients surviving five years or longer following operation will differ from its true value only by random variation. Consequently, the sample size should be large enough so that the estimates have sufficient precision. For example, it is not very meaningful to state that a surgical procedure is successful in 75 per cent of cases when the number of cases is four. The true percentage of successful cases could vary markedly from 75 per cent. However, the figure is very meaningful when the number of cases is 400. Should the numbers observed be small and consequently the precision be too low, then no real conclusions can be drawn from the investigation. When too large a study has been undertaken and the results are more precise than needed, then experimental resources have been wasted. Appropriate size of sample is therefore an important consideration.

In any study, *the range of validity of the conclusions* depends markedly on the particular set of units used and the variety of conditions investigated. Additional uncertainty is involved when the conclusions are to be applied to new conditions or units. For example, the results of a surgical study involving only young patients may not be applicable to older patients. Ideally the units in an experiment should be chosen from a well-defined population of units by an appropriate statistical procedure for sampling. In a clinical study this is difficult to achieve. However, the patients in the study should be representative of a well-defined type. Strictly interpreted, the results apply only to the types of patients involved in the study. Therefore, it is desirable to examine a broad range of conditions since the wider the range of conditions investigated, the greater the confidence in extrapolating conclusions. This is very important when the study is designed to determine the applicability of a treatment to a wide class of patients and less so when the primary object is to gain insight into a particular treatment.

It is generally *important to keep a study relatively simple.* Too many factors should not be investigated in any one study. When a study is a cooperative venture involving a number of institutions, it is especially important to have a simple design to avoid problems of misinterpretation at the various institutions. Sometimes, a portion of the professional group are involved more in planning and analysis, and others are involved more in carrying out the studies. In such experiments, with delegation of responsibility, it is especially important that the design be simple. Having such a design implies that the analysis will also tend to be simple. Unforeseen problems are more likely to have an adverse effect on an investigation of complex design than one of simple design.

GENERAL PRINCIPLES OF ANALYSIS

The most informative summaries of data are simple descriptive statistics such as the percentage of patients responding to treatment, the average or median length of disease-free interval following operation, percentage of smokers among cases of bronchogenic carcinoma, etc. An estimate of the variability of the average value(s) selected should also be given, such as the standard error of a proportion or the standard error of an average value. Simply reporting average values ± 2 standard-error limits will give a good indication of how precisely effects have been estimated in a study. The larger the sample size, the more narrow the limits and consequently, the better the estimate of average effect.

In retrospective or prospective studies concerned with comparisons of average values, it is often desirable to decide whether differences observed in the sample represent real differences in the population from which the samples were derived or whether the differences were likely to have arisen from chance fluctuations. To reach a decision, two hypotheses are set up: a null hypothesis which asserts that there is no real difference in the average values and an alternative hypothesis * which asserts a real difference in average values.

To test a null hypothesis, the assumption is made that it is true. Then the probability of obtaining a sample difference as great or greater than that observed is calculated, assuming the difference arose because of chance alone. When the probability is very low, say 5 per cent or less, the investigator will tend to reject the null hypothesis and declare that some real difference exists in sample proportions, averages, etc. This probability is called the significance level, and it is generally set at 5 per cent or 1 per cent. When the probability of obtaining the observed data is rather high, say of the order of 20 per cent or more, the investigator declares there is not sufficient evidence present in the data to reject the null hypothesis. The data cannot prove the null hypothesis; however, they can be consistent with it. Reasonable interpretations of the results of significance tests are as follows:

Significance Level of Data	Interpretation
Less than 1 per cent	Very strong evidence against the null hypothesis.
1 per cent to 5 per cent	Moderate evidence against the null hypothesis.
More than 5 per cent and less than 10 per cent	Suggestive evidence against the null hypothesis.
10 per cent or more	Little or no real evidence against the null hypothesis.

---

* See appendix i for definitions and details of calculations.

III

RETROSPECTIVE STUDIES*

AIMS AND ADVANTAGES

THE AIM OF A RETROSPECTIVE STUDY is usually (1) to discover associations existing between the presence of a disease such as bronchogenic carcinoma and the possession of some characteristic such as smoking cigarettes; and (2) also the term may be used for retrospective studies in which different regimens of treatment are compard for their efficacy. The former is "one in which the determination of association of a disase with some factor is based on unusually high or low frequency of that factor among diseased persons."† The latter type of study is nearly always uncontrolled, since cases may not be comparable with respect to age, severity of disease, etc.

Retrospective studies are appealing because the data to be used are at hand, but they have acquired a certain stigma because desirable information is frequently incomplete in available records. However, it is often surprising how much of the clinical picture may be reconstructed from the past by careful inquiry, linkage of sources one to another,[9] and proper construction of the retrospective study itself. A retrospective study may even be the method of choice when all pertinent considerations are compared.

Retrospective studies have certain advantages relative to prospective studies. First, the sample size required is much smaller, and the study is easier to plan and execute than a prospective study. For example, to study the relationship between carcinoma of the urinary bladder and smoking, a very large sample of smokers and nonsmokers would be required in a prospective study; and a substantial follow-up period would be necessary before many cases would be expected in the smoking and nonsmoking groups. However, it would be relatively simple to locate existing cases of carcinoma of the urinary bladder in a hospital population and compare their smoking experience with a control group. Consequently, the retrospective study is a natural method of approach for an investigator with limited resources, although selection of an appropriate group for control is laden with hazards.

---

* A complete discussion of the retrospective study in the field of cancer epidemiology is given by Lilienfeld, Pederson, and Dowd,[35] and the analysis of various types of retrospective study is given by Mantel and Haenszel.[37]

† Mantel and Haenszel.[37]

The problems involved in obtaining an unbiased comparison are similar in both types of retrospective studies. In a prospective study various events are studied during a specified interval of time, but a retrospective study requires reliance on mnemonic and recorded evidence for the occurrence of past events. The results from prospective studies are generally more likely to be unbiased and therefore convincing to a disinterested audience than results from retrospective studies, and a finding from a single retrospective study is infrequently convincing alone, requiring additional confirmatory studies. When proper adjustments are made so that groups of individuals are as comparable as possible in all respects except the one under study, such as a surgical procedure, the retrospective type of study may be useful in assessing the results of treatment. In addition, promising leads for prospective studies may be suggested by the results.

An investigation may be a simple comparison of cases with the disease or receiving treatment and those cases used as controls, popularly known as a case-control study. A refinement is the retrospective study of matched samples. Also adjustments for differences in a factor between cases and controls may be advantageous.

The determination of an association does not necessarily imply that possession of a factor is causal in its relationship to the occurrence of a disease. However, further study to determine the strength of the association, specificity, consistency, dose-response relationship, and possibly a confirming prospective study may enable the investigator to assert that there is a causal relationship between presence of the factor and presence of the disease.

The exemplary retrospective study of Snow showing the relationship between the source of drinking water and distribution of deaths from cholera was performed over 100 years ago. The work of Holmes on puerperal fever had the advantage of a well-defined segment of the hospital population for study. More recent examples of retrospective studies leading to conclusions of great significance are those relating smoking to disease. Early work by Wynder and Graham [49] and by Doll and Hill [20] was followed by numerous studies culminating in the "Report on Smoking and Health" prepared by the Surgeon General's Committee on Smoking and Health.[43] Some of these investigations constitute good illustrations of problems encountered and techniques for solving them. Therefore it is profitable to examine some of the data on mortality ratios for bronchogenic carcinoma in smokers and nonsmokers as an example of a study relating the onset of a disease with a specific factor. The relationship between operative mortality and hepatic function in a study of end-to-side and side-to-side portacaval shunts will then be used to illustrate methods for handling comparison of data on two methods of surgical management.

SIMPLE RETROSPECTIVE STUDY OF CASES AND CONTROLS

Data published by Doll and Hill [20] given in the following table illustrate a simple type of retrospective study of cases and controls.

TABLE 1

STUDY OF BRONCHOGENIC CARCINOMA IN SMOKERS AND CONTROLS

	No. of Smokers	No. of Nonsmokers	Total	Per Cent Smokers
Males with Bronchogenic Carcinoma	647	2	649	99.7
Male Control Patients	622	27	649	95.8
Total	1,269	29	1,298	

From these key data Doll and Hill concluded "that smoking is a factor, and an important factor, in the production of carcinoma of the lung." The 649 males with bronchogenic carcinoma from twenty hospitals in London were from a larger group of 2,370 notifications of patients with cancer between April 1948 and October 1949. As far as possible, each case of bronchogenic carcinoma was matched by interviewing a patient of the same sex, within the same five-year age group, and in the same hospital at or about the same time. Since the authors did not analyze the data in a way to take advantage of the matching and presented it as two independent samples, one of the cases and one of controls, it is presented here as a simple case-control study rather than a study of matched samples.

After cases and controls were interviewed to ascertain their status as smokers or nonsmokers and various other data related to their exposure to atmospheric pollution, careful confirmation of the information was obtained by reviewing the diagnosis and comparing cases and controls with respect to social class and place of residence. A sample of individuals was interviewed a second time to determine the consistency of the interviewing with respect to the determination of smoking status. Also, the smoking experience of those incorrectly thought to have carcinoma of the lung at the time of interview was found to be similar to that of controls rather than that of patients with the disease, eliminating a possible tendency on the part of the interviewers to exaggerate the experiences with smoking of those with carcinoma.

These data illustrate a well-controlled retrospective study. The cases and controls were matched by age and sex and were as comparable as possible with respect to other variables. Possible sources of bias in the selection of cases and interviewing were investigated, and the authors [20] conclude that "it is not reasonable, in our view, to attribute the results to any special selection of cases or to bias in recording. In other words, it must be concluded that there is a real association between carcinoma of the lung and smoking."

The statistical test on which this statement is based is the chi-square test of association in 2×2 tables.* The null hypothesis tested by the chi-square test is that the true percentage of individuals with the characteristic, smoking, is the same in the case and control groups. The hypothesis alternative to the null hypothesis can be either one- or two-sided. In the former case, the alternative hypothesis is that the true percentage of persons with the characteristic is greater in the group of cases than in the controls. The alternative that it is smaller also may be selected by the investigator in another example as more appropriate, but one or the other alternate hypothesis must be chosen for the one-sided test, not both. In the two-sided case, the alternative hypothesis is that the true percentage with the characteristic is different when the case and control groups are compared. The difference can be either greater or smaller.

In a prospective study, representative groups of persons having and not having the characteristic are selected, and the percentage in each group who have the disease or develop it during the designated interval of time is determined. This yields a true rate. An aim in a retrospective study of disease is to determine whether the probability of having or incurring a disease during a specified period of time is related to possession of some characteristic. Two groups respectively presumed to be representative of persons who do and who do not have the disease are used to determine the percentage in each group who have the characteristic. Rather than determine the percentage of smokers and nonsmokers who have cancer of the lung, the percentage of persons with and without bronchogenic carcinoma who are smokers is determined. This yields a relative frequency. Using certain assumptions,[14] it is possible to deduce the rates from the knowledge of the relative frequencies and results from retrospective studies are usually given in terms of relative risks. In the example used, interest resides in the relative risk of developing bronchogenic carcinoma between those who did and did not smoke.

A measure of the relative risk for having the disease for the simple retrospective study of cases and controls is defined as

$$\frac{\text{Proportion of persons having the characteristic and the disease}}{\text{Proportion of persons not having the characteristic and having the disease}}$$

The data analyzed by Doll and Hill indicate that the risk† of developing bronchogenic carcinoma for smokers is fourteen times greater than the risk for nonsmokers.

---

* The general arrangement for the test and the details of the calculations for another example are given in appendix ii, 1.

† The method of calculating relative risk is given in detail in appendix iii, 1.

The chi-square test of association is also a test of whether or not the relative risk is unity in a retrospective study. Hence, if the chi-square test indicates a significant statistical association, then it also means that the relative risk is significantly different from unity.* For these data chi-square $(\chi^2) = 20.32$ and $P<.01$ which is statistically significant and very strong evidence against the null hypothesis.

An example of a retrospective study in which two surgical procedures are compared is adapted from data published by Child.[12] The percentage of postoperative deaths following end-to-side portacaval shunts is compared to that following side-to-side portacaval shunts for the treatment of portal hypertension. Data for the end-to-side procedures are given for the period 1952-1963 and for the side-to-side procedure the period is 1959-1963. Hence, part of the time the procedures are being studied concurrently, although cases are not randomized, and part of the time the only comparison possible is a retrospective one. The data are contained in Table 2.

TABLE 2
MORTALITY FOLLOWING TWO TYPES OF SHUNTS
FOR PORTAL HYPERTENSION

	Postoperative Death			Per Cent Mortality
	Yes	No	Total	
End-to-side Shunt (1952-63)	22	107	129	17
Side-to-side Shunt (1959-63)	7	30	37	19
Total	29	137	166	

Clearly, there is little overall difference in the percentage of postoperative deaths between the two procedures. However, the importance of hepatic functional reserve in relation to postoperative deaths becomes apparent when the percentage of postoperative deaths (4 per cent in 95 patients) in patients with minimal or moderate impairment is compared to the percentage in patients with advanced impairment (53 per cent in 34 patients). Arranging data for operative procedures into subclasses of patients according to deranged hepatic function is obtained in Table 3.

Although the number of patients is small in some groups and sources of bias may be present, these data suggest that the percentage of postoperative deaths following the end-to-side shunt is lower in patients with minimal or moderate impairment in hepatic function and higher in patients with advanced impairment than the respective percentages following the side-to-side shunt.

---

* The problem of finding confidence limits for the relative risk from a retrospective study is discussed by Cornfield[14] and Lilienfeld, Pederson, and Dowd.[35]

TABLE 3

EFFECT OF DERANGED HEPATIC FUNCTION ON MORTALITY
FOLLOWING OPERATIONS FOR PORTAL HYPERTENSION

Impairment in Hepatic Function	*End-to-Side*				*Side-to-Side*			
	Postoperative Death			*Per Cent Death*	*Postoperative Death*			*Per Cent Death*
	Yes	*No*	*Total*		*Yes*	*No*	*Total*	
Minimal or Moderate	4	91	95	4	2	21	23	9
Advanced	18	16	34	53	5	9	14	36
Total	22	107	129	17	7	30	37	19

The appropriate statistical test for comparing the mortality following two surgical procedures is the chi-square test.* It is also appropriate when the data are subclassified according to hepatic function, assuming that the differences in postoperative mortality are in the same direction for all levels of impaired hepatic function. The data can be summarized in a 2×2 table or several 2×2 tables when the data are subclassified. The x^2 test shows a significant difference ($P<.05$) when the mortality from either type of operation in those with advanced hepatic impairment is compared to that for those with minimal or moderate impairment. Another interesting comparison is the mortality after the two types of operations for those with impaired function which appears possibly to be a real difference. However, the chi-square test indicates there is no statistically significant difference in the results of the two types of operations when the liver is greatly damaged ($P>0.4$) or minimally to moderately damaged ($P>.5$).

RETROSPECTIVE STUDY OF MATCHED SAMPLES

In a study of matched samples, individual cases are matched with individual controls for various factors such as age, sex, socioeconomic status, etc. that are considered to have a possible association with the disease. When a large number of factors are used in matching or when each factor has many levels, it is difficult to find a mate for every case; therefore it is best to have a limited number of levels of each factor. For example, five- or ten- rather than one-year intervals of age are ordinarily chosen.

Studies with matched samples are less subject to bias than when cases and controls are taken from different populations; and the precision of comparisons between cases and controls is increased, since the comparisons are accomplished within relatively homogeneous groups. The increase in precision is dependent upon the existence of a high correlation between the matching characteristic and the disease or variable being studied. Al-

---

* Appendix ii.

though these are advantages, it should be recognized that the numbers of factors for which matching is feasible usually is rather small.

Lilienfeld[34] interviewed a sample of the adult population of Buffalo, New York to determine whether cigarette smokers differed from nonsmokers with respect to emotional status and other characteristics. One index of emotional status was the answer to whether the respondent ever felt like smashing things for no good reason. In the entire sample, 903 cigarette smokers were matched with 903 nonsmokers with respect to age (twelve age groups), sex, race (white and nonwhite) and social class (four quartiles). Thus, there were $12 \times 2 \times 2 \times 4 = 192$ possible subgroups for each individual. The replies of the 903 pairs of smokers and nonsmokers about their emotional status may be classified as follows:

TABLE 4

REPLIES TO QUESTION ABOUT FEELING LIKE SMASHING THINGS FOR NO APPARENT REASON BY MATCHED PAIRS OF SMOKERS AND NONSMOKERS

| | *Smokers* | | |
Nonsmokers	*Sometimes or Often*	*Never*	*Total*
Sometimes or Often	30	111	141
Never	192	570	762
Total	222	681	903

The design of this table, although straightforward, may not be evident at first glance. The replies of each pair of individuals are allocated to respective cells in the table according to whether both members of the pair sometimes or often felt like smashing things for no good reason, neither member of the pair ever felt this way, or the members differed in their feelings about smashing things. Thus, 570 pairs of individuals among the 903 never felt like smashing things. This should be distinguished from tabular presentations for simple studies of cases and controls. If the study had involved independent samples of smokers and nonsmokers, the available data would be in the margins of the table, indicating that 141 nonsmokers and 222 smokers out of 903 sometimes or often felt like smashing things. In the study of matched samples, pairs of individuals are classified with respect to the presence or absence of the characteristic under study.

The chi-square test for this type of study* shows that a significantly higher percentage of cigarette smokers compared with nonsmokers sometimes or often feel like smashing things for no good reason. Lilienfeld noted that smokers were significantly different (P<.02) from nonsmokers in sixteen out of thirty-one items; in each instance the responses of smokers were excessive in the direction that might be considered neurotic. How-

---

* Appendix ii, 2 contains calculations more in detail.

ever, he stated that "the degree of difference between smokers and non-smokers was not sufficient to account for the high degree of association between cigarette smoking and bronchogenic carcinoma and therefore could not influence the causal inference derived from this association, though it might be sufficient to explain the association of cigarette smoking with peptic ulcer and coronary-artery disease."

The relative risk is a convenient summary statistic to use in presenting the results of a study of matched samples. In the study under discussion, the risk of feeling like smashing things for no good reason is R = 1.73 times greater for smokers compared to nonsmokers;[*] and the chi-square test[†] indicates that the risk is significantly different from unity (P<.05).

STUDIES ADJUSTING FOR DIFFERENCE IN ONE FACTOR IN CASES AND CONTROLS

Wynder and Graham[49] compared the smoking habits of 605 male patients with epidermoid or undifferentiated bronchogenic carcinoma to those of 780 individuals from the population in a general hospital. No attempt was made to match patients by age and consequent distributions by age differed between cases and controls, as shown in Table 5.

TABLE 5

SMOKING HABITS OF PATIENTS WITH BRONCHOGENIC CARCINOMA COMPARED TO THOSE IN A POPULATION FROM A GENERAL HOSPITAL GROUPED BY AGE

Age Group	Males with Bronchogenic Carcinoma			Controls			Cases and Controls		
	Smokers	Non-smokers	Total	Smokers	Non-smokers	Total	Smokers	Non-smokers	Total
30-39	13	1	14	126	20	146	139	21	160
40-49	105	0	105	148	16	164	253	16	269
50-59	254	4	258	189	21	210	443	25	468
60-69	184	2	187	137	23	160	322	25	347
70-79	40	1	41	75	25	100	115	26	141
Total	597	8	605	675	105	780	1272	113	1385

Only two categories are recorded for the characteristic studied—smoker or nonsmoker.[‡]

The chi-square test may be used for testing whether smokers have a higher risk of developing bronchogenic carcinoma, adjusting for differences in distribution of ages.[§] The assumption is made that the associa-

---

[*] Appendix iii 2, contains details of the calculations.

[†] Appendix ii, 2 contains calculations more in detail.

[‡] Mantel and Haenszel[37] discuss the more general case in which the characteristic studied is at more than two levels. For example, many studies have recorded levels of smoking by numbers of cigarettes smoked per day.

[§] See appendix ii, 3 for details of calculations.

tion, if present, is consistent over the various decades of age. The test would not be appropriate, for example, if younger smokers were less likely to develop bronchogenic carcinoma, whereas older smokers were more likely to develop the disease for the same duration of exposure.

TABLE 6

RELATIVE RISK FOR BRONCHOGENIC
CARCINOMA IN SMOKERS

Age Group	Relative Risk
30–39	2.062
40–49	. . . . . .*
50–59	7.057
60–69	15.542
70–79	13.331
Total	11.608

* The relative risk is undefined, since no non-smokers in the 40-49 age group developed bronchogenic carcinoma.

The relative risk* of developing bronchogenic carcinoma for smokers compared with nonsmokers is significantly higher in each age group, except 40-49 where it is undefined. The relative risk for all smokers regardless of age, which is known as the crude relative risk, is a summary relative risk involving no adjustment for differences in the age distributions. It is 11.6 and significantly higher for smokers than nonsmokers.

Two summary measures of relative risk recommended by Mantel and Haenszel[37] provide adjustments for differences in age and essentially are weighted averages of the relative risks within each age group. One overall measure of relative risk, designated R_1, is an adjusted crude relative risk and the value is 8.97 for this study. The other measure of overall relative risk, designated R, is that preferred by Mantel and Haenszel[37] and in this case is 10.37. Therefore all measures of summary relative risk are substantially greater than unity, suggesting that smokers have about a ten-fold risk of developing bronchogenic carcinoma compared with nonsmokers. Since the three measures of overall relative risk yield similar values in this example, any one of three methods used for weighting individual relative risk will not be misleading and can be chosen with confidence. A chi-square test† may be used to test whether the overall relative risks R or R_1 are significantly in excess of one.

PROBLEMS IN RETROSPECTIVE STUDIES

The outstanding difficulty in a retrospective study of cases and controls is obtaining a set that are representative of their respective popula-

* Calculations are explained in appendix iii, 3.

† The test is explained and the calculations carried out in appendix ii, 3.

tions. Usually, case and control groups are selected from hospital populations or consecutive autopsies. The question then arises whether an association found between the occurrence of some disease and the possession of a characteristic arose because of a real difference between cases and controls or because of selective factors. Although it is not possible to perform a retrospective study free of all bias, sources of bias should be carefully assessed for their possible influence on the results and eliminated as nearly as possible so that they are negligible or not sufficient to explain associations that are identified. Several retrospective studies may be required to confirm a real association when there is a possibility of bias.

Bias in the selection of patients autopsied is illustrated by Pearl's study of the possible association between cancer and tuberculosis.[41] Using data from the first 7,500 autopsies performed at the Johns Hopkins Hospital, Pearl compared the percentage of patients with tuberculous lesions among 816 individuals with cancer and 816 control patients matched for age, sex, race, and date of autopsy. In the control group, 16 per cent of patients had tuberculous lesions, whereas only 6.6 per cent had such lesions in the group with cancer. A difference of this magnitude was also evident when the patients were studied separately for white males and females and nonwhite males and females. Since other checks on the data showed the same negative association, Pearl concluded that tuberculosis was antagonistic to cancer.

Unfortunately the control group autopsied provided a biased estimate of the prevalence of active tuberculous lesions among all noncancerous individuals, since a large number of individuals in the control group actually died from tuberculosis and the group necessarily had a higher prevalence of tuberculous lesions than all of the individuals living without cancer.[47] Carlson and Bell[11] used only those who died from cardiac disease as a control group and found approximately the same percentage of individuals with tuberculous lesions both in the group with cancer and the group with cardiac disease. Therefore, they could not confirm that tuberculosis was antagonistic to cancer. Pearl reached a false conclusion because his control group provided a biased estimate of the prevalence of tuberculous lesions in a living population.

Usually retrospective studies of cases and controls are conducted with hospitalized patients. Berkson[6] has demonstrated the possibility of falsely obtaining an association between diseases or between a characteristic and a disease because of different probabilities of admission to the hospital for individuals with the disease, for those without the disease, and for those with the characteristic. Since an observed association may be a reflection of the selective biases for admission to a hospital, it is incumbent on an investigator to judge how much weight should be given to the possible influence of such biases. For example, the characteristic under investigation may be associated with another characteristic causally related to the disease.

When hospitalized patients are used as controls, some protection against bias can be built into the design of the study. For example, control groups may be drawn from a variety of diseases diagnosed on admission and the control groups then examined to see whether the frequency of the characteristics observed among the control groups differs substantially or not. This provides protection against two sources of bias: (1) finding an association between a characteristic and a disease when the association is really related to the disease group from which the controls were obtained and (2) failure to detect an association because both the study and control groups were associated with the suspected factor. For example, patients dying from coronary-artery disease would not constitute suitable controls for a study of the relationship between smoking and bronchogenic carcinoma, since the investigator might conclude that smoking was not related to either, when in fact it appears related to both.

If patients are being interviewed, it is usually advantageous to include several items in the questionnaire for which data from the general population are available. This enables the investigator to check on the representative nature of the control group. The identity of the cases and controls should be unknown to the interviewer to guard against possible bias. Alterations of diagnoses subsequent to interview can provide a useful test for bias. Sometimes certain factors are known to be related to disease such as age, sex, and economic level. In this situation, such factors should be matched between disease and control groups. Unfortunately, the group of cases is preselected in terms of disease, so the investigator usually has no control over the number of cases in any particular grouping for age or sex. If the structure of the sample of cases is known, the simplest method of matching is to arrange patients in the population of controls according to the structure in the population of cases. Random samples of the same size found in the sample with disease are then taken at each level. Alternatively, cases and controls can be matched individually as described in the section on studies of matched samples. When a characteristic is used for matching, it is eliminated as an independent variable for study.

INFERENCES FROM RETROSPECTIVE STUDIES

If a retrospective study results in an association being found between the characteristic and occurrence of a disease, this association could be spurious, indirect, or causal. If it can be demonstrated that an association could have resulted from a bias in the selection of the case or control groups, then the observed association is likely to be spurious. If the possible biases have been investigated and found not sufficient to account for the degree of association found, then it may be concluded that the association is indirect or causal.

An association between a characteristic and a disease may be indirect because of the presence of a second factor that is common to both the characteristic and the disease. For example, the observation that patients with bronchogenic carcinoma have peptic ulcer more often than those without the disease probably arises because each of these diseases is related to cigarette smoking rather than because of a direct association between the two diseases. The recognition of the possibility of this type of association provides the remedy. Thus, those with the disease and the characteristic should be studied for the possibility of a factor common to both.

Some investigators declare a causal relationship whenever evidence appears that possession of some characteristic(s) forms part of a chain of events increasing the chance of developing a disease, and absence of these characteristic(s) lessens the frequency of the disease. Other investigators require a more rigorous definition such as evidence that a factor is both a necessary and a sufficient condition for a disease before it can qualify as a cause. However, declaration of causality only when both of these last two requirements are met seems unduly stringent for biological studies because of the existence of multiple causative factors. For example, the tubercle bacillus is a necessary but not a sufficient condition for tuberculosis.

The performance of experiments using patients and controls, determining etiologic mechanism(s) of the disease, and acquisition of additional epidemiologic evidence are useful for pursuing likely causal relationships. A prospective study may be undertaken in which a possible etiologic characteristic is randomly allocated to the first group and withheld from the second, although this type of study will not often be possible in human populations. If a prospective study can be done, it eliminates the possibility of an indirect association as the explanation for any observed difference between the incidence of the disease in the experimental and the control group. A second possibility is to conduct an experiment to determine whether cessation of habit or lessening of exposure to an environmental factor of possible etiologic significance results in a decrease in incidence of a particular disease.

Direct experimentation is desirable to determine etiologic mechanism(s) and constitutes the best kind of evidence that a characteristic is causal. The hazard of transferring conclusions from experiments with animals is well known, but more ingenious use of human tissues *in vitro* fortunately is gradually reducing these difficulties.

Additional evidence supporting the causal significance of a statistical association may consist of examination of aspects of the association previously unexplored or different types of studies permitting a choice between the causality and indirect association. The first approach should determine the strength of the association. If all cases of a particular disease possessed a characteristic and none of the controls did, the causal hypothesis would be substantiated. Failing that, a high relative risk should be required. If an association is specific for a particular disease, the causal hypothesis is more likely. Conversely, relationship with the particular disease is less likely to be causal when the associated factor is found to be related to many diseases. The greater the number of causal agents involved in producing a particular disease, the weaker will be the association between any single factor and the disease. When a characteristic is causally related to a disease, then the risk of developing the disease should be related to the degree of exposure to the characteristic, and the observation of such dose-response relationship increases the likelihood of a causal hypothesis.

The distribution of the suspected etiologic factor in the population should be determined in terms of age, sex, race, and other characteristics. The distribution of the disease in the population according to the same characteristics should then be determined. If these distributions are consistent, the plausibility of the causal hypothesis will be increased, since it would be very unlikely for an indirect association to operate in the same way in a variety of subgroups in the population. The possibility of a causal relationship between the characteristic and the disease is strengthened if an association is repeatedly found in many studies, but particularly when carried out in different groups of populations and different countries.

The performance of an experiment in a human population or the determination of the mechanism by which the disease is produced provides the strongest evidence concerning a cause and effect relationship. Studies yielding additional epidemiologic evidence serve the purpose of supporting either the hypothesis for causal or indirect association.

IV

PROSPECTIVE STUDIES

A PROSPECTIVE STUDY MAY BE PLANNED (1) to investigate the relationship between the occurrence of a disease or a medical event and the presence of some factor in the population, or (2) to determine the effectiveness of a surgical procedure or therapeutic regimen administered to diseased persons. There is a crucial distinction between these types of studies. In the former, the observer has no control over the distribution of individuals among groups. For example, it is not possible to assign one set of individuals to a smoking group and a second set to a nonsmoking group if the effect of smoking is being studied. In a clinical trial, assignment of an individual to a specified management is the prerogative of the investigator.

The aim of a prospective study of the first type is usually to confirm associations uncovered in a retrospective study and has many of the hazards of the latter. Problems shared by both types of studies include setting up an adequate control group and obtaining representative data. Interesting conclusions can be drawn from prospective studies when comparisons are made between matched groups of individuals such as those with similar range of age, duration of symptoms, social habits, etc. However, more cogent conclusions about causal relationship to clinical management can be drawn from the second type of experiment designated as the clinical trial. Therefore, primary consideration will be devoted to the clinical trial.

The types of clinical trial are delineated in Figure 1. Clinical trials may be planned for a wide variety of treatments including surgical procedures, regimens of drugs, and radiotherapeutic schedules. A clinical trial does not test a procedure or drug itself; it does test effectiveness of a procedure when carried out in a particular manner for a certain type of patient. When management is changed even slightly, a very different order of effectiveness may emerge. For example, response may differ greatly according to the schedule or route of administration of a drug.[45] The connotation implied by the term, "clinical trial," should not be restricted to the comparative, or phase-III, trial. Although most reports of clinical trials consist of comparative trials, studies prior to comparative trials may be of equal or greater importance.

PHASE-I STUDIES

The early or phase-I trial is an exploratory investigation of several procedures or regimens used with different types of patients in search of one

[23]

TYPES OF CLINICAL TRIAL FOR A SURGICAL PROCEDURE OR NEW THERAPEUTIC REGIMEN

SEQUENCE OF CLINICAL TRIALS

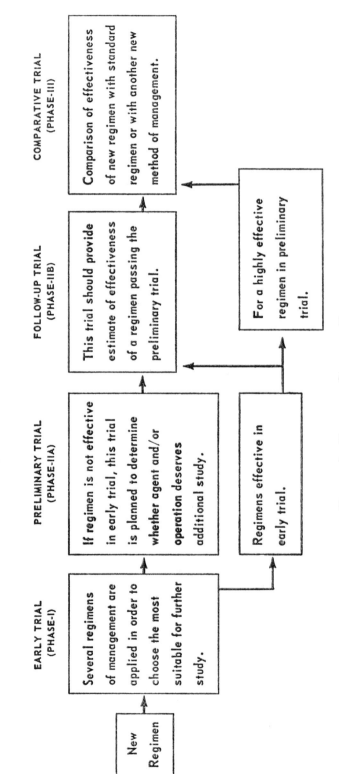

FIGURE 1. TYPES OF CLINICAL TRIAL

that can be used in additional studies. A patient in a drug trial is started at a particular dosage level, and then the amount of drug is increased gradually until a level of dosage is achieved that is toxic or effective in the patient. Eventually, a regimen of dosage is chosen that can be tolerated by a majority of patients. The type of operation or dosage of drug to be used initially may be selected from antecedent experiments with laboratory animals.[24]

No single formal design for a phase-I study can be recommended. Proposals for such plans have been made, but the knowledge and intuition of the investigator is much more important than a specific experimental design. A measure of response in a clinical trial is usually a simple criterion, such as decrease in tumor volume to one half the starting level. However, changes in all relevant characteristics of the patient should be used in choosing the management deserving additional study. If no effect of management has been noted in phase I, a phase-IIA trial may be undertaken. For treatment that has been effective, a follow-up study should be conducted (phase IIB).

PHASE-II TRIALS

Preliminary Study (Phase IIA)

Usually the purpose of a preliminary trial is to yield evidence for a choice between two points of view: (1) the regimen is unlikely to be effective in X percentage of patients or more, or (2) the regimen could be effective in X percentage of patients or more. If the purpose of the study can be summarized in this manner, it can be accomplished with a relatively small number of patients. Table 7 provides the size of sample necessary to make one of the above two decisions at given levels of rejection error. The rejection error is the chance of failing to undertake an additional trial, when studies should have been continued.

TABLE 7

SAMPLE SIZE (n) REQUIRED FOR A PRELIMINARY TRIAL (PHASE IIA)
IN TERMS OF GIVEN LEVELS OF THERAPEUTIC EFFECTIVENESS
AND REJECTION ERROR (β)

Permissible Rejection Error (β)	*Level of Therapeutic Effectiveness (Per Cent)*									
	5	10	15	20	25	30	35	40	45	50
5 Per Cent	59	29	19	14	11	9	7	6	6	5
10 Per Cent	45	22	15	11	9	7	6	5	4	4

When a regimen of 20 per cent effectiveness or more is of interest and a rejection error of 5 per cent acceptable, then a trial with fourteen patients should be undertaken. For a regimen 20 per cent effective or more, there would be more than a 95 per cent chance that one or more successes would be obtained in fourteen consecutive cases. Thus, when one observed fourteen consecutive failures, the first decision above would be made. The chance of having rejected a regimen of 20 per cent effectiveness or more is less than 5 per cent. If one or more successes were observed, the second decision above would be justified and study of additional patients required to establish the effectiveness of the regimen.

The phase-IIA trial is designed so that the minimum possible number of consecutive failures is observed before study of a regimen is halted. Investigators often include only three or four patients and terminate treatment when no responses are observed. This practice invites great risk for missing an effective regimen of management. For example, the chance of missing a regimen as highly effective as 50 per cent is one in eight when only three patients are studied.

The definition of therapeutic effectiveness requires careful assessment. In diseases for which previous procedures or drugs have been completely ineffective, the definition may pose no serious difficulties, and any objective benefit to the patient may be classified as a therapeutic effect. But if transient regressions or partial benefits are frequently observed, it is reasonable to require pronounced objective improvement in the patient's disease as evidence for therapeutic effectiveness. The requirement of objective measurements with limits for determining effectiveness prevents classification of biological variations in the disease or minor benefits as successes. When very effective management already exists, a phase-IIA trial will not be very useful, since nearly all regimens will pass the preliminary trial and require further study. On the other hand this type of trial will eliminate regimens having little or no effectiveness.

Follow-up Study (Phase IIB)

When a regimen has passed a phase-IIA trial or has been sufficiently effective in a phase-I trial, then a follow-up trial is recommended in order to provide a precise estimate of the effectiveness of a particular regimen.

An estimate of true effectiveness is the proportion of patients in the sample who are treated successfully, designated $\hat{p}$, and the precision of this estimate is measured by its standard error.

$$\text{Standard Error } (\hat{p}) = \sqrt{\frac{p\,(1-p)}{n}}$$

where $\hat{p}$ = proportion of treatment successes in sample
(proportion must be between 0 and 1)
p = true proportion (unknown) of successes following treatment
n = number of patients.

Since p is always unknown, $\hat{p}$ is substituted for p to obtain an estimate of the standard error. The largest possible standard error($\hat{p}$) is obtained when p = 0.5; therefore the standard error ($\hat{p}$) is less than or equal to $0.5/\sqrt{n}$.

A reasonable requirement for a follow-up study is that it should yield an estimate of therapeutic effectiveness with a specified relative precision. Relative precision is the ratio of the standard error($\hat{p}$) to $\hat{p}$. It is roughly the proportional variation in the estimate of $\hat{p}$. When the relative precision is zero, there is no variation in the estimate of $\hat{p}$.

For a regimen effective in early trial that is to be studied in a follow-up trial, the number of patients required to achieve a specified relative precision is given in Table 8. When a relative precision of .20 is desired, this would correspond to a standard error of .02 if the true proportion of effectiveness were .10, but would correspond to a standard error of .08 if the true proportion of effectiveness were .40. Usually, more precision is required for a small proportion than for a large proportion of patients treated effectively.

TABLE 8

NUMBER OF PATIENTS REQUIRED FOR SPECIFIED
RELATIVE PRECISION *

Relative Precision	.10	.15	.20	.25	.30	.35	.40
No. of Patients (n) Required	100	45	25	16	12	9	7

$$* \text{ Relative Precision} = \frac{\text{Standard Error } (\hat{p})}{\hat{p}} = \sqrt{\frac{(1-\hat{p})}{n\hat{p}}}$$

A simple rule of thumb with a slight but conservative error may be used to estimate the number of patients required in the follow-up trial. The number in the follow-up trial should make the total number (those in the preliminary trial plus those in the follow-up trial) sufficiently large to achieve a specified relative precision. Thus, when fourteen patients have been studied in a preliminary trial (phase IIA) and the relative precision required is .20, then eleven additional patients are required in the follow-up trial.

THE COMPARATIVE CLINICAL TRIAL (PHASE III)

The role of the comparative trial in clinical research has elicited great interest and discussion. In Atkins' view,[4] the controlled clinical trial has led to a number of new discoveries and has been of great importance ever since it was introduced in Great Britain in the 1930's by Hill.[31] This view has been disputed by Hoffer,[32] who has stated that this type of trial has led to no new developments (at least in mental health research) and in fact has tended to stifle investigation of new ideas. Perhaps its value is intermediate to these views.

Part of the difference in viewpoint is semantic in that some writers refer to the clinical trial without specifying the type. Consequently, some investigators have embarked on rather large-scale comparative clinical trials when a preliminary or follow-up trial was the type actually needed. Others have studied different methods of managing patients during different chronological periods and then compared the methods of management as if a comparative trial were undertaken. The first consideration of those planning a clinical trial should be to determine where the work with a particular agent or method of management should be located in the sequence of clinical trials given in Figure 1. It should not be undertaken when a regimen or procedure is still being actively developed so that the likelihood of change within a relatively short time is great.

Important aims of a comparative clinical trial are: (a) to select the better treatment for future use in management of patients, (b) to estimate the effectiveness of each regimen of treatment (or the difference in effectiveness) with some degree of precision, and (c) to estimate the effects of treatment with given precision and to select the better treatment. The primary purpose of the trial should be considered carefully. For example, a trial in which the number of patients studied is the minimum necessary to reach a decision as to which is the better treatment would probably be chosen if the purpose were that given in (a), but it would not be appropriate for (b).

As far as possible, a comparative clinical trial should be set up so that the only difference between groups is the actual treatment(s) received. This requires comparability in the way patients are entered into the investigation, managed during study, and analyzed when the study is completed. If these rules are not followed, the results may be inconclusive or interpreted erroneously. To achieve comparability of patients at time of entry, they should be randomized by some device such as the use of appropriate tables of numbers. A description of techniques for randomizing patients to two or more regimens of treatment is given in Appendix vi with tables of random digits. In order to avoid bias in the selection of patients for study, the investigator should not be aware of the outcome of randomization beforehand.

Failure to randomize properly may lead to erroneous conclusions if bias is sufficiently great. For example, more patients with severe myocardial infarction were included in one than in the other group when the results of treatment with two anticoagulants were compared in a study by Achor et al.[1] Myocardial infarction was severe in forty-two patients out of 122 treated with heparin, whereas only twenty-one out of 122 had severe myocardial infarction in the group treated with warfarin. As a result, treatment with heparin would be presented in an unfavorable position no matter what hypothesis was to be tested because of a relatively high proportion of severely ill patients receiving the treatment. Therefore any investigator sufficiently prejudiced in favor of therapy with heparin to the extent that he entered patients with severe myocardial infarction on that therapy would likely see the results of the study the reverse of his expectations. The bias in the randomization would make it more likely that warfarin would be the treatment that appeared superior in the study.

It is also important to manage patients the same way within each regimen. If some or most investigators in a group have a strong preference for one of the treatments, they may maintain patients on it longer in the presence of toxicity or other deleterious effect in search of a response. This could seriously alter the results in favor of the treatment originally preferred. One solution to this problem is to use a double-blind study. For example, medication may be prepared in identical capsules so that the physician is unaware of the treatment administered. Another is to require objective evidence that a patient is deteriorating before he can be dropped from study or have the regimen changed. When such a decision cannot be divorced from subjective evaluation, a second investigator's opinion may be required. When operations are included in the protocol, double-blind designs obviously do not apply, although entry of a given case into the study may be randomized in prearranged fashion.

Finally, all patients entered should be analyzed the same way when study is completed, especially when subjective responses are being evaluated. A prejudiced investigator can influence whether or not a patient is classified as a responder or not. A remedy for this type of problem is a blind evaluation of cases. That is, the evaluator should be unaware of what treatment the patient has received when he makes his determination of response.

Assuming that there is comparability in the way patients are entered, managed while the study is in progress, and analyzed when the investigation is completed, additional factors deserving consideration are the use of a control group, the categories of patients for study, end-points in the analysis of the study, and statistical considerations.

Considerations in the Planning of Comparative Trials

Use of a Concurrent Control Group

An issue in planning a comparative trial is whether or not a concurrent control group should be used or whether historical controls suffice. For example, suppose a study is to be planned comparing length of survival following operation or operation plus chemotherapy in the treatment of glioblastoma multiforme. Substantial data exist in reports of Roth and Elvidge [44] and Frankel and German [23] giving length of survival following operation, to suggest that these data provide historical control. However, the data were collected over a long period of time (30 years or more), and it is likely that patients entered in a study now would have somewhat different operative and supportive care than those reported. Certain factors in these studies favored longer survival, namely, being young, female, and having a total resection. There is no assurance that a study done now would have similar proportions of patients in each of these categories as those previously reported. In any clinical trial, candidates for study are selected from among the total patients seen, whereas historical surveys generally give results for consecutive patients and it is impossible to know how the factors used for selection affect survival. Questions about a biased comparison are much less likely to arise from skeptics when two treatments to be compared are given concurrently.

A case for using historical controls can be made when a clinical trial is to follow a previous one from which the control cases are derived, provided there is reasonable likelihood that results in control groups will be the same in both studies. Even so, it is usually better to include some patients in the control treatment to check whether results are similar to those obtained previously.

Categories of Patients for Study

Patients can always be divided into subcategories. For example, in carcinoma of the colon, they may be divided by location of lesions, stage of lesions (I-IV), previous management, duration of symptoms, etc. A clinical trial designed to yield the results of two methods of treatment may be planned (1) to compare the overall effects of the two treatments ignoring subcategories or (2) to compare the two treatments within each subcategory. The second type of trial will be larger than the first by a factor equal to the number of subcategories.

A trial of the first type should be planned when it is reasonable to expect the same order of difference between treatments to be observed in each subcategory. For example, one might be concerned with the proportion of patients having a complete remission or disappearance of their malignant disease in relation to the stage at the time of management. If treatment A has an 80 per cent rate of response in stages I and II and a 40 per cent rate of response in stages III and IV, and a new treatment B is expected to be effective in 10 per cent more patients than A in all stages, it would be appropriate to have a trial of the first type. If the difference in percentage effectiveness between A and B is expected to differ by stage, even in a different direction, then a trial of the second type should be planned. A clinical investigation of the second type may be regarded as a group of separate clinical trials, one for each subcategory.

Definition of Response

The definition of a response must be precise for a clinical trial, and selection from possible end-points must be a judicious part of the design. A few possible choices of response are length of time to recurrence of disease following surgery, proportion of patients having complete remission of their disease after six weeks of therapy, proportion of patients surviving five years or more, and length of survival following treatment. Response also may be designated as a mathematical function of several variables.* The choice of a primary end-point determines, in pronounced fashion, the type of trial, the range of interpretations which emerge at the conclusion, and possibly the length of the trial.

Several factors should be considered in choosing an end-point. Generally a quantitative variable, such as survival time, will lead to a more efficient trial than a qualitative one, such as proportion surviving five years. Survival time is clearly a meaningful variable, but its use is complicated because patients may die of causes unrelated to their disease, may receive treatments other than those in the trial before death, or may survive too long for a clinical trial of reasonable duration. Time to recurrence or extension of disease can be a useful variable because it is always shorter than survival time and is frequently correlated with survival time. However, a disease-free status may be difficult to define, verification during the course of the study may be complex, and freedom from disease may not be well correlated with survival. For a particular trial, various end-points should be considered for their meaningfulness and the length of trial implied. Gehan[26] found that a particular clinical trial, under various stratagems of entering patients, could last 2.4 to 10 years, depending upon the purpose and choice of end-point—disease-free interval or survival. The primary purpose of the trial, the number of patients anticipated, and length of trial required to achieve the purpose are all related to end-point(s) chosen.

Statistical Considerations

Statistical considerations are related to the philosophy of the investigator(s) planning the trial as well as tests for significance. The merits of the frequentist, Bayesian, and likelihoodist viewpoints are still actively being investigated, and a complete discussion of each is beyond the scope

---

* See Grizzle[30] for discussion.

of this text. However, a few remarks are in order about the distinguishing characteristics of each.

In a frequentist trial, the investigator specifies the level of significance (α), the value of the desired power ($1\text{-}\beta$), the difference between treatments important to detect (in terms of percentage of responders or in terms of a quantitative difference), and some estimate of the variability of response in each treatment group. The level of significance (α) is the chance of a false-positive statement, i.e., the trial ends with the conclusion that there is a real difference between treatments when in fact there is none. The chance of a false negative statement is designated as β, i.e., the trial ends with the conclusion that there is no difference between treatments when, in fact, there is. The chance that the clinical trial will declare as statistically significant a given real difference in response is ($1\text{-}\beta$) or the power. Comparative clinical trials are formal procedures in which frequentists set up an hypothesis and an alternative and specify the chance for a false-positive error (α) and the chance for a false-negative error (β). The hypothesis is then accepted or rejected on the basis of statistical significance of observed differences in results of treatment. However, a consensus is emerging * that very rarely is a clinical trial simply a test of a single hypothesis, but out of the complexity of a trial emerges information about response, toxicity, etc. In summarizing this view, Greenhouse [19] suggests that ". . . the classical precepts of the specification of the two types of possible error and their relationship to the determination of sample size should serve as a guide to help make decisions in the planning stages of the study. As such, this framework can be most useful. But it should neither bind the investigator or the statistician in the analysis of the data nor in the information obtainable from the data."

Although the frequentist viewpoint is adopted in this paper, alternative philosophies for interpreting data from clinical trials should be mentioned briefly. Recently, Bayesian methods,† named after the Reverend Mr. Thomas Bayes whose theorem appeared in 1763, have been reexamined. These methods require utilization of prior information about treatments being examined, modified by the likelihood of the results observed in the trial to obtain posterior probabilities about the relative merits of the two treatments. The distinction between Bayesian and frequentist methodologies is the formal use of prior information for making an inference in the former. Subjective Bayesians postulate the odds favoring each treatment intuitively. An objective Bayesian utilizes only information based upon available data concerning the treatments.

---

* See Cutler *et al.*[19] for discussion.

† Both subjective and objective Bayesian viewpoints are discussed by Plackett.[42]

The likelihoodist * draws inferences as the trial progresses based on the likelihood of the data favoring a specific treatment and uses neither significance tests nor prior information. In sequential trials, termination of the investigation depends on the data accumulated rather than conditions specified in advance as in the frequentist's approach.

The approximate number of patients needed in trials planned from Bayesian and likelihoodist viewpoints may be computed from advance estimates of relative merits of the treatments examined.[15, 26]

Other Factors

Limiting factors in the design of a clinical trial are its length and the clinical and analytical resources along with the number of patients available. Although no specific rules can be given, interest and enthusiasm for a clinical trial often are decreasing functions of time. Therefore long clinical trials should be undertaken only when duration is carefully assessed and justified. An estimated number of patients and the approximate length of the trial should be determined in advance so that one can decide whether or not the resources are sufficient. If not, the purpose of the trial should be reexamined and a more limited trial undertaken. For example, it would be better to do a study of consecutive cases rather than to start a controlled clinical trial that had little or no chance of being finished satisfactorily.

When prior information is scanty, a feasibility study will reveal whether the methods visualized *a priori* are useful in actual practice within a short span of time. Unless the preliminary work suggests that the investigation should be abandoned, the study can proceed with greater assurance of success, alterations having been made consonant with the results of the feasibility study.

Size of Sample in Comparative Clinical Trials

The size of sample for a particular comparative clinical trial depends upon the purpose of the study (estimation, selection, selection and estimation); the statistical philosophy (frequentist, Bayesian, or likelihoodist); and certain considerations appropriate to the particular study. The viewpoint in the following discussion is that of the frequentist, and size of sample will be discussed for trials with selection of the better treatment as the primary purpose.

It is assumed that two regimens of management are to be compared and a trial to select the better of the treatments is to be planned. A sequential trial or a trial involving a fixed number of patients given each regimen

---

* A good discussion of the likelihoodist viewpoint may be found in the paper by Plackett.[42]

may be chosen. For the latter, two percentages and/or two average values may be compared, and the investigator must choose a difference between treatments (in percentages or average values) that he considers important to detect, tolerable levels of false positive and false negative error, and an estimate of the variability of the difference in response.

Sequential Clinical Trials

In a sequential trial of a type given by Armitage, who has published many sequential schemes,[3] patients are paired and each member receives

TABLE 9 A

NUMBER OF PATIENTS NEEDED IN AN EXPERIMENTAL AND A CONTROL GROUP FOR A GIVEN PROBABILITY OF OBTAINING A SIGNIFICANT RESULT (ONE-SIDED TEST)

Smaller Proportion of Success (P_1)	Larger Minus Smaller Proportion of Success (P_2-P_1)													
	.05	.10	.15	.20	.25	.30	.35	.40	.45	.50	.55	.60	.65	.70
.05	330	105	55	35	25	20	16	13	11	9	8	7	6	6
	460	145	76	48	34	26	21	17	15	13	11	9	8	7
	850	270	140	89	63	47	37	30	25	21	19	17	14	13
.10	540	155	76	47	32	23	19	15	13	11	9	8	7	6
	740	210	105	64	44	33	25	21	17	14	12	11	9	8
	1370	390	195	120	81	60	46	37	30	25	21	19	16	14
.15	710	200	94	56	38	27	21	17	14	12	10	8	7	6
	990	270	130	77	52	38	29	22	19	16	13	10	10	8
	1820	500	240	145	96	69	52	41	33	27	22	20	17	14
.20	860	230	110	63	42	30	22	18	15	12	10	8	7	6
	1190	320	150	88	58	41	31	24	20	16	14	11	10	8
	2190	590	280	160	105	76	57	44	35	28	23	20	17	14
.25	980	260	120	69	45	32	24	19	15	12	10	8	7	..
	1360	360	165	96	63	44	33	25	21	16	14	11	9	..
	2510	660	300	175	115	81	60	46	36	29	23	20	16	..
.30	1080	280	130	73	47	33	24	19	15	12	10	8	..	..
	1500	390	175	100	65	46	33	25	21	16	13	11	..	..
	2760	720	330	185	120	84	61	47	36	28	22	19	..	..
.35	1160	300	135	75	48	33	24	19	15	12	9	..	..	..
	1600	410	185	105	67	46	33	25	20	16	12	..	..	..
	2960	750	340	190	125	85	61	46	35	27	21	..	..	..
.40	1210	310	135	76	48	33	24	18	14	11	..	..	..	..
	1670	420	190	105	67	46	33	24	19	14	..	..	..	..
	3080	780	350	195	125	84	60	44	33	25	..	..	..	..
.45	1230	310	135	75	47	32	22	17	13	..	..	..	..	..
	1710	430	190	105	65	44	31	22	17	..	..	..	..	..
	3140	790	350	190	120	81	57	41	30	..	..	..	..	..
.50	1230	310	135	73	45	30	21	15	..	..	..	..	..	..
	1710	420	185	100	63	41	29	21	..	..	..	..	..	..
	3140	780	340	185	115	76	52	37	..	..	..	..	..	..

Upper Figure: Test of significance at .05 for α, power equals .8 for $(1-\beta)$.
Middle Figure: Test of significance at .05 for α, power equals .9 for $(1-\beta)$.
Lower Figure: Test of significance at .01 for α, power equals .95 for $(1-\beta)$.

one of the two treatments by random allocation. Responses of paired patients are compared, and entry of patients continues until a decision is made about which treatment (depending on difference between treatments) is superior. The boundary point for this decision is defined by the sequential plan chosen in advance of the trial. Therefore, sequential trials depend not only on the information accumulated but also on the plan chosen in advance of the trial. An attractive feature of such a plan is the fixed upper limit to the number of patients needed. Also, the sample sizes

TABLE 9 B

NUMBER OF PATIENTS NEEDED IN AN EXPERIMENTAL AND A CONTROL GROUP FOR A GIVEN PROBABILITY OF OBTAINING A SIGNIFICANT RESULT (TWO-SIDED TEST)

| Smaller Proportion of Success (P_1) | Larger Minus Smaller Proportion of Success (P_2-P_1) | | | | | | | | | | | | | |
	.05	.10	.15	.20	.25	.30	.35	.40	.45	.50	.55	.60	.65	.70
.05	420	130	69	44	31	24	20	16	14	12	10	9	9	7
	570	175	93	59	42	32	25	21	18	15	13	11	10	9
	960	300	155	100	71	54	42	34	28	24	21	19	16	14
.10	680	195	96	59	41	30	23	19	16	13	11	10	9	7
	910	260	130	79	54	40	31	24	21	18	15	13	11	10
	1550	440	220	135	92	68	52	41	34	28	23	21	18	15
.15	910	250	120	71	48	34	26	21	17	14	12	10	9	8
	1220	330	160	95	64	46	35	27	22	19	16	13	11	10
	2060	560	270	160	110	78	59	47	37	31	25	21	19	16
.20	1090	290	135	80	53	38	28	22	18	15	13	10	9	7
	1460	390	185	105	71	51	38	29	23	20	16	14	11	10
	2470	660	310	180	120	86	64	50	40	32	26	21	19	15
.25	1250	330	150	88	57	40	30	23	19	15	13	10	9	..
	1680	440	200	115	77	54	40	31	24	20	16	13	11	..
	2840	740	340	200	130	92	68	52	41	32	26	21	18	..
.30	1380	360	160	93	60	42	31	23	19	15	12	10	..	..
	1840	480	220	125	80	56	41	31	24	20	16	13	..	..
	3120	810	370	210	135	95	69	53	41	32	25	21	..	..
.35	1470	380	170	96	61	42	31	23	18	14	11	..	..	..
	1970	500	225	130	82	57	41	31	23	19	15	..	..	..
	3340	850	380	215	140	96	69	52	40	31	23	..	..	..
.40	1530	390	175	97	61	42	30	22	17	13	..	..	..	..
	2050	520	230	130	82	56	40	29	22	18	..	..	..	..
	3480	880	390	220	140	95	68	50	37	28	..	..	..	..
.45	1560	390	175	96	60	40	28	21	16	..	..	..	..	..
	2100	520	230	130	80	54	38	27	21	..	..	..	..	..
	3550	890	390	215	135	92	64	47	34	..	..	..	..	..
.50	1560	390	170	93	57	38	26	19	..	..	..	..	..	..
	2100	520	225	125	77	51	35	24	..	..	..	..	..	..
	3550	880	380	210	130	86	59	41	..	..	..	..	..	..

Upper Figure: Test of significance at .05 for α, power equals .8 for $(1-\beta)$.
Middle Figure: Test of significance at .05 for α, power equals .9 for $(1-\beta)$.
Lower Figure: Test of significance at .01 for α, power equals .95 for $(1-\beta)$.

are on the average smaller than those required by equivalent plans with fixed size of sample.

Many successful sequential trials have been conducted using one of the plans given by Armitage. These plans are useful when the purpose is to select the better of two treatments, when there is an ethical reason for wishing to stop the trial as soon as a significant difference is achieved, when estimation of treatment effects is a secondary consideration, and when it is convenient to pair patients on the two treatments. A sequential plan will not be very suitable when some of these conditions are not met and when response to treatment can only be determined after a substantial follow-up period. In the latter case, pairs of patients would continue to be entered into study when there were already many pairs of patients on the study in which the response status could not yet be determined. Limitations of space do not permit additional elaboration of these methods.

Trials with Fixed Size of Sample

A clinical trial involving a fixed number of patients is generally simple to design, simple to administer, and, since some estimate is usually available for the number of patients that can be entered per year, the length of the trial can be predicted within reasonable limits. These trials usually involve more patients and last longer than equivalent sequential trials but better estimates of the effectiveness of each treatment can be made because more patients are entered. The numbers of patients given should be taken as guidelines for the numbers required.

TRIALS WITH FIXED SIZE OF SAMPLE FOR COMPARING TWO PERCENTAGES. When responses are qualitative (success or failure, response or no response, etc.), the appropriate size of sample in each of two groups may be determined from tables 9A or 9B adapted from Cochran and Cox.[13] The number of patients in experimental and control groups is given in table 9A for a one-sided test (experimental is better than control group) and in table 9B for a two-sided test (either treatment may be superior to the other). The two-sided test may be used for comparing two proposed treatments or experimental and control management.

As an example, suppose the rate of response to the control treatment is 25 per cent and a clinical trial is to be designed to detect whether an experimental treatment is 20 per cent more effective than the control treatment. Examination of table 9A shows that sixty-nine patients are required in both groups for a significance level of .05 and a power of 0.8 in a one-sided test. Sizes of sample required for two-sided tests (table 9B) are always larger than those required for one-sided tests with the same specifications. Before choosing a final size for the sample, the investigator(s) should examine the number of patients required for differences in percentage response and different levels of power and statistical significance. A choice can then be made in accord with overall aims.

TRIALS WITH FIXED SIZE OF SAMPLE FOR COMPARING TWO AVERAGE VALUES. When response to treatment is measured quantitatively rather than qualitatively and the measured response follows the normal distribution approximately, the sample size required may be determined by reference to an appropriate table[13, 46] if the values for true differences in response, power, significance, and variability are assigned properly. If the data contain a substantial proportion of very large or small observations, then the skewed data may be transformed to achieve more symmetry by taking logarithms. Data frequently skewed are survival times (usually some long survivors) and blood counts (usually some high counts).

First the investigator must decide the value of δ, the true difference between the effect(s) of treatments he regards as important. The probabilities of obtaining a significant result (power or $1-\beta$) should usually be in the neighborhood of .80, .90, or .95. A required level of significance (α) must be chosen also. Finally, an investigator must supply an estimate of the true variability of the observations (either σ_d for the case of paired samples or σ_p for the case of two independent samples). Estimates of variability * are usually obtained from pilot studies planned for this purpose or from knowledge gained in previous experiments.

When the investigator has specified a value for the difference to be detected (δ); the desired probability ($1-\beta$) for obtaining a significant result when the true difference is δ; the significance level (α) of the test (which may be one- or two-sided); and an estimate of variability (σ_d for paired samples or σ_p for independent samples), then the following table adapted from Snedecor and Cochran[46] may be used to determine size of sample.

TABLE 10

MULTIPLIER TO BE USED IN DETERMINING SIZE OF SAMPLE FOR A COMPARATIVE CLINICAL TRIAL WITH SIZE FIXED

Power $(1-\beta)$	Two-sided Test			One-sided Test		
	Level of Significance (α)			Level of Significance (α)		
	.01	.05	.10	.01	.05	.10
.80	11.7	7.9	6.2	10.0	6.2	4.5
.90	14.9	10.5	8.6	13.0	8.6	6.6
.95	17.8	13.0	10.8	15.8	10.8	8.6

* Calculations for estimates of variability are explained in appendix iv.

Sample size n = (multiplier from table) $\dfrac{\sigma_d^2}{\delta^2}$ for paired samples　　　(i)

Sample size n = (multiplier from table) $\dfrac{2\sigma_p^2}{\delta^2}$ for independent samples　　　(ii)

As an example, suppose the effects of two treatments on hemoglobin level are being compared in a two-sided test. The investigator designs an experiment in which individuals are to be randomized into two independent samples and hemoglobin levels are to be measured before treatment and two hours after receiving treatment. The average change in level of hemoglobin considered important to detect is a difference (δ) of 1 g/100 ml. The variability in hemoglobin level (σ_p) is estimated to be 1.5 g/100 ml. The desired significance level (α) for the two-sided test is .05 and the probability ($1-\beta$) of declaring the given difference to be significant is .90. Then, the appropriate multiplier from the table is 10.5, and the required sample size in each group (from formula ii above) is

$$n = \frac{(10.5)\ (2)\ (1.5)^2}{1^2} = 47.25$$

Since sample size thus obtained should always be rounded upward, 48 individuals would be required.

In most experimental situations, investigators cannot be completely precise about specifications. Therefore, the sample size should be determined for several sets of specifications and a final choice made consistent with the resources available. Constructing a table such as the following may be useful in making a final choice of sample size:

TABLE 11

SIZES OF SAMPLE FOR SPECIFIC TRIAL CALCULATED
FOR SEVERAL RESPECTIVE SETS OF SPECIFICATIONS

Power $(1-\beta)$	Difference in Hemoglobin Levels (g/100 ml)			
	0.5	1.0	1.5	2.0
.80	143	36	16	9
.90	189	48	21	12

A final choice of a sample of 48 individuals can then be made with full knowledge of the sample sizes implied by other specifications. The size required increases when the level of significance is decreased, when the probability of detecting a difference as significant is increased, and when the difference in effect between treatments is decreased. Sample sizes are smaller for one-sided than comparable two-sided tests.

ANALYSIS OF DATA

Comparison of Two Percentages

It is common in clinical trials to obtain data for two treatment groups so that each patient can be classed as a responder or nonresponder, success or failure, etc. A chi-square test is then used to determine whether or not there is a real difference in the proportion of responders in the two groups.

The following example from the paper by Fisher *et al.*[21] is a useful example illustrating a comparison of percentages. The incidence of recurrence in premenopausal patients with four or more positive nodes found at the time of radical mastectomy is collated on the basis of whether or not adjuvant chemotherapy was administered.

TABLE 12

RECURRENCE OF MAMMARY CARCINOMA
FIVE YEARS OR LESS AFTER TREATMENT

Management Adjuvant to Radical Mastectomy	Recurrent Carcinoma			
			Total	
	Positive	Negative	Number	Per Cent
Thio-TEPA	15 (17.9)	8 (5.1)	23	65
Placebo	31 (28.1)	5 (7.9)	36	86
Total	46	13	59	78

Numbers expected appear in parentheses.

These data are from a large-scale investigation of the role of adjuvant therapy with Thio-TEPA * at the time of radical mastectomy in the treatment of carcinoma of the breast. In the Thio-TEPA group, 65 per cent of the premenopausal patients with four or more positive nodes had recurrence of the disease within five years after operation compared with 86 per cent of patients in the placebo group. The numbers in the table are those observed in the study, with those expected in parentheses, assuming that there was no real difference in the percentage of patients recurring in each group. Were there no difference in rates of recurrence, the recurrence rate for all patients, 78 per cent, would be applicable in each group. The expected numbers are obtained by assuming this rate of recurrence for the 23 patients in the Thio-TEPA group and the 36 patients in the placebo group.

In this case, the null hypothesis is that the percentage of patients having a recurrence in the Thio-TEPA group is the same or higher than that in the placebo group. The alternative hypothesis is that the true percentage

---

* Triethylenethiophosphoramide.

of patients having a recurrence is lower in the group of patients receiving Thio-TEPA. The observed data show that 21 per cent fewer patients had recurrence in the Thio-TEPA group compared with the placebo group. A chi-square test * is used to test the null hypothesis. The test is appropriate when the total sample is 20 or more and the expected values in each cell are 5 or more. In this case, the value of chi-square is 2.38 and the level of significance between 6 and 7 per cent. Therefore these data provide suggestive evidence that the true percentage of patients having a recurrence in the Thio-TEPA group is lower than that in the placebo group. For tables in which the size of sample is less than 20 and for tables in which the expected values are small, Fisher's exact test is recommended.[†]

Comparison of Two Average Values

PAIRED DATA. Student's test [‡] may be used to test whether a real difference exists between two average values obtained from paired data. It is relatively insensitive to departures from the assumption required for its validity that the data be normally distributed and each observation have the same variability. The following data are from Student's original paper.[22]

TABLE 13

ADDITIONAL HOURS OF SLEEP GAINED BY THE
USE OF TWO TYPES OF TREATMENT

Patient	Treatment A	Treatment B	Difference $(B-A)$
1	0.7	1.9	1.2
2	−1.6	0.8	2.4
3	−0.2	1.1	1.3
4	−1.2	0.1	1.3
5	−0.1	−0.1	0
6	3.4	4.4	1.0
7	3.7	5.5	1.8
8	0.8	1.6	0.8
9	0	4.6	4.6
10	2.0	3.4	1.4

The null hypothesis is that the true average difference in hours of sleep gained is zero. The alternative hypothesis is that the true difference is greater or less than zero (a two-sided test). The t value [§] is statistically significant at the one-per-cent level. Therefore these data provide very strong evidence that the two treatments differ in their sleep-producing qualities and the difference favors treatment B. The estimate of the average

---

* The calculations are explained in appendix ii, 1.

† This test and chi-square tests for more complicated sets of data are given by Maxwell.[39]

‡ The t test was developed by W. S. Gosset in 1908. He worked for the Guiness Brewery in Dublin and published his research under the pseudonym of Student because of company policy.

§ Calculations are included in appendix iv, 1.

difference ($\bar{d}$) in hours of sleep gained through treatment B compared to treatment A is 1.58 hours with standard deviation (s_d) $= 1.23$ hours.

UNPAIRED DATA. A t test is used when the difference between average values in two independent samples is to be tested. The number of individuals in each sample need not be equal. As an example, suppose two types of operative procedures are being compared in a clinical trial, and the investigator wishes to test whether the true average age of patients having each type of operation is the same. In a sense, this is a test of the randomization procedure, since the randomization of patients should insure that patients are comparable with respect to age, sex, and other factors possibly related to response to treatment.

TABLE 14

TEST FOR RANDOMIZATION IN UNPAIRED DATA

Treatment 1		Treatment 2	
Average Age ($\bar{x}_1$)	$= 58$ Years	Average Age ($\bar{x}_2$)	$= 55$ Years
Number of Patients (n_1)	$= 20$	Number of Patients (n_2)	$= 18$
Standard Deviation (s_1)	$= 6.7$ Years	Standard Deviation (s_2)	$= 8.0$ Years

In this case, the null hypothesis is that there is no real difference in average ages. The natural alternative hypothesis is two-sided: there is a difference in true average ages between treatment groups. Calculation of the t test for this case* indicates that the probability of such an observed difference in average ages is greater than .20 and therefore the data provide no evidence that the true average ages differ.

Analysis of Data for Survival Time

The response recorded in clinical studies is often some measure of time, such as survival time. Survival time can be defined in various ways: length of life from onset of symptoms, diagnosis, or treatment; time free of disease following operation; time to recovery following spinal-cord injury; time to improvement from start of specified treatment; etc. Data for survival time often include some censored[†] survival times, illustrated by the following typical set.

Survival Time (Months)

$$2, 2, 3, 3+, 4, 5, 5+, 6, \ldots$$

The times 3+, 5+ are censored; these individuals were still alive when last observed at 3 and 5 months respectively. Since censored data complicate the analysis of a set of survival times, the methods selected for discussion

---

* See appendix iv.

† The designation that a survival time is censored means that the individual is alive at the time of analysis or was alive when last seen.

are valid when they are present. Note that it is not possible to calculate an average survival time when there are censored times. The average of the above figures, ignoring the censored values, gives a minimum average survival time. Descriptive, or graphical, methods and methods not dependent on assuming particular forms of theoretical survival distribution will be discussed rather than analytical methods such as choosing a model to fit the data and estimating parameters for distributions of survival time.

A small sample of survival times without censored observations provides an example for analysis.

Survival Time (in Months) of Men Following Initial
Pulmonary Metastasis from Osteogenic Sarcoma
(n = 11 patients)

11, 13, 13, 13, 13, 13, 14, 14, 15, 15, 17

Unless the theoretical form of the distribution for survival time is known from previous data, only simple descriptive measures are available such as:

Median survival time = survival time of the patient in the
middle of the ordered observations

The middle patient is $(n + 1)/2$ where n is the number of patients.

Median = survival time of the $(11+1)/2 = $ 6th patient = 13 months

Range = longest survival − shortest survival = $17 - 12 = 5$ months

A simple abridged method for estimating standard deviation and standard error of survival time which is valid in small samples $(n \leqslant 12)$ has been given by Mantel.[36] The estimates are:

$$Standard\ Deviation \approx \frac{Range}{\sqrt{n}} = \frac{5}{\sqrt{11}} = 1.5$$

and

$$Standard\ Error\ of\ Mean \approx \frac{Range}{n} = \frac{5}{11} = .455$$

These values can be used to obtain rapid estimates of variability from small samples and are very close to those calculated from the longer formulae,* 1.4 and .443, respectively.

Figure 2 is an example of a survival curve often known as a survivorship function. The proportion surviving is 1.00 when all the patients are alive and decreases to zero when all individuals have died. The median survival time $(t_{med.})$ can be read from the graph and is the value at which one-half the patients are still alive.

---

* See appendix i.

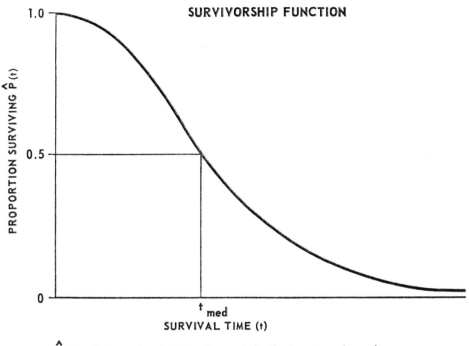

$\hat{P}(t) = $ Estimated probability that an individual survives beyond t.

FIGURE 2. SURVIVORSHIP FUNCTION

The survival times of 36 patients with glioblastoma multiforme may be used as an example. The patients were divided into two groups; the experimental group contained 21 patients who had operations and chemotherapy for their disease, and the control group contained 15 patients who had operative procedures only for their disease. The data are those available about one year after the start of the study and are used for purposes of illustration only.*

TABLE 15

SURVIVAL TIMES WITH CENSORED OBSERVATIONS FOR
PATIENTS WITH GLIOBLASTOMA MULTIFORME

Group	No. of Patients	Survival Time (Weeks)*
Experimental	21	1, 2, 2, 2, 2+, 6, 8, 8, 9, 9+, 13, 13+, 16, 17, 22+, 25+, 29, 34, 36+, 43+, 45+
Control	15	0, 2, 5, 7, 7+, 11+, 12, 19+, 22+, 30+, 35+, 39+, 42, 46, 54

   * A + value means that the patient was alive at last report; all are rounded to the nearest whole number of weeks.

   * The study is being conducted by the Brain Tumor Study Group, jointly sponsored by the National Cancer Institute and the National Institute of Neurological Diseases and Blindness.

The survival times of the patients in the experimental and control groups appear in Table 15.

Various estimates of median survival time can be calculated and are tabulated below.

TABLE 16
MEDIAN SURVIVAL TIMES FOR PATIENTS WITH
GLIOBLASTOMA MULTIFORME

Group	No. of Patients	Median Survival Time		
		Minimum	*Maximum*	*Estimated*
Experimental	21	13	17	16
Control	15	19	54	34

To calculate the minimum median, it is assumed that all patients with plus values died immediately after the last report. For the maximum median, it is assumed that patients with plus values survived beyond the longest survival time recorded. In both cases, the survival time in the middle of the ordered observations is taken as an estimate of the median. The difference between the minimum and the maximum median is an indication of how well the sample median has been determined. When there is a small difference between the minimum and the maximum, the sample median is well bracketed, whereas a large difference indicates that the sample median is not well determined. In the above data, the sample median is fairly well bracketed in the experimental group, but not in the control.

The survivorship function is estimated according to a method* given by Kaplan and Meier,[33] a procedure yielding $\hat{P}(t)$, the estimated proportion of individuals alive at time t after the start of the study. This estimate can be made when censored and failure times are present in the set of observations. Survival curves for the patients with glioblastoma multiforme are given in Figure 3. The estimated median survival time is 16 weeks in the experimental group and 34 weeks in the control group. Other percentiles of survival time may be read directly from the chart. When a large sample of survival times is available, a life-table method† can be used to estimate the survivorship function.[7, 18, 27] The life-table method requires that the observations be grouped into intervals, and the estimate of survivorship will depend, to some extent, on what intervals are chosen for grouping. The estimate of Kaplan and Meier and that from the life-table give nearly the same results in large samples of about 50 or more.

---

* A computer program is available for calculating $\hat{P}(t)$.

† This method is often called the Berkson-Gage method.[7]

However, the former method can be used in relatively small samples and does not require any arbitrary grouping of data.

It is clearly more informative to construct a survival curve rather than a one-year, five-year, ten-year, or other survival proportion, since the proportion of individuals surviving to any given year may be read from

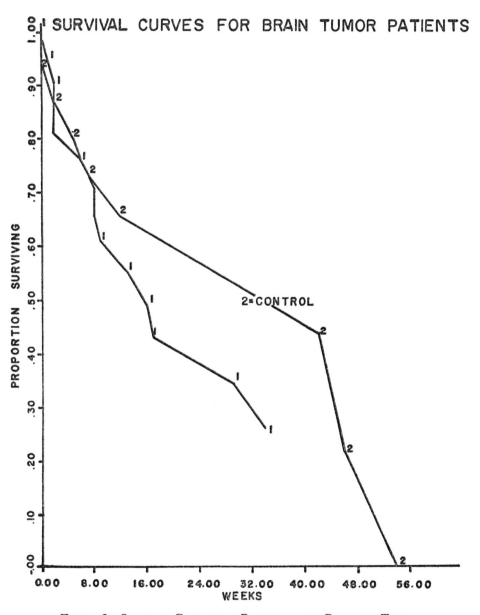

FIGURE 3. SURVIVAL CURVES FOR PATIENTS WITH CEREBRAL TUMORS

the curve. Also, survival proportions in two groups may be nearly equivalent for any given year when the entire survival experience is quite di-
vergent. One group may have a high proportion of early deaths and fewer
deaths thereafter and the other group fewer early deaths and a higher
proportion occurring later. Survival curves demonstrate this difference,
whereas reporting only survival proportions may obscure it.

A modification of the Wilcoxon* test[25] is appropriate for testing the
difference between two survival curves whether or not censored observations are present. It is also appropriate whatever the true forms of survival
curve in the two groups. In the test of the difference between survival
curves for glioblastoma multiforme, the null hypothesis is that there is
no real difference between survival curves for experimental and control
groups. The alternative hypothesis is that survival is longer in the experimental group. The statistic used in the generalized Wilcoxon test, W, has
a probability of greater than 0.3 by chance alone. This indicates that these
data provide no real evidence for a difference in survival curves favoring
the experimental group.

---

* Details of the calculations for this test are given in appendix v.

BIBLIOGRAPHY

1. ACHOR, R. W., *et al.* (Cooperative Study): Sodium heparin *versus* sodium warfarin in acute myocardial infarction, *JAMA, 189*(6):555-562, 1964.
2. ANSCOMBE, F.: Sequential medical trials, *J Amer Statis Assn, 58*(302):365-387, 1963.
3. ARMITAGE, P.: Sequential Medical Trials. Great Britain, Blackwell Scientific, 1960, pp. 105.
4. ATKINS, H.: Conduct of a controlled clinical trial. *Brit Med J, 2*:377-379, 1966.
5. BACON, R.: De *erroribus medicorum*, translated by E. T. Withington. In *Essays on the History of Medicine Presented to Karl Sudhoff*. London, Oxford U P, 1924, pp. 139.
6. BERKSON, J.: Limitations of the applications of fourfold table analysis to hospital data, *Biomet Bull, 2*:47-53, February, 1946.
7. BERKSON, J., and GAGE, R. P.: Calculation of survival rates for cancer. *Proc of the Staff Meetings of the Mayo Clinic, 25*:270-286, 1950.
8. BRINKLEY, D., and HAYBITTLE, J. L.: Results of treatment of carcinoma of the breast, *The Lancet, 1*:86-90, 1959.
9. BURDETTE, W. J.: *Methodology in Human Genetics*. San Francisco, Holden Day, pp. 436, 1964.
10. BULL, J. P.: The historical development of clinical therapeutic trials, *J Chronic Dis, 10*(3):218-248, 1959.
11. CARLSON, H. A., and BELL, E. T.: Statistical study of occurrence of tuberculosis and cancer in 11,195 postmortem examinations, *J Cancer Research, 13*:126-135, 1929.
12. CHILD, C. G., III: *The Liver and Portal Hypertension*. Philadelphia, Saunders, pp. 231, 1964.
13. COCHRAN, W. G., and COX, G. M.: *Experimental Designs*. New York, Wiley, 1957, pp. 611.
14. CORNFIELD, J.: A method of estimating comparative rates from clinical data. Applications to cancer of the lung, breast, and cervix, *J Nat Cancer Inst, 11*(6): 1269-1275, 1951.
15. CORNFIELD, J.: A Bayesian test of some classical hypotheses with applications to sequential clinical trials, *J Amer Statis Assn, 61*:577-594, 1966.
16. COX, D. R.: *Planning of Experiments*. New York, Wiley, pp. 308, 1958.
17. CROW, J. F.: A chart for the χ^2 and t distribution, *J Am Statis Assoc, 40*:376, 1945.
18. CUTLER, S. J., and EDERER, F.: Maximum utilization of the life table method in analyzing survival, *J Chronic Dis, 8*(6):599-712, 1958.
19. CUTLER, S. J.; GREENHOUSE, S. W.; CORNFIELD, J., and SCHNEIDERMAN, M. A.: The role of hypothesis testing in clinical trials, *J Chron Dis, 19*:857-882, 1966.
20. DOLL, R., and HILL, A. B.: Smoking and carcinoma of the lung: Preliminary report, *Brit Med J, 2*:739-748, 1950.
21. FISHER, B.; RAVDIN, R. G.; AUSMAN, R. K.; SLACK, N. H.; MOORE, G. E., and NOER, R. J.: Surgical adjuvant chemotherapy in cancer of the breast, *Ann Surg, 168*:337-356, 1968.
22. FISHER, R. A.: *Statistical Methods for Research Workers*, 13th ed., Edinburgh, Oliver and Boyd, 1963, pp. 339.

23. FRANKEL, S. A., and GERMAN, W. J.: Glioblastoma multiforme: Review of 219 cases, *J Neurosurg, 15*:489-503, 1958.

24. FREIREICH, E. J.; GEHAN, E. A.; RALL, D. P.; SCHMIDT, L. H., and SKIPPER, H. E.: Quantitative comparison of toxicity of anticancer agents in mouse, rat, hamster, dog, monkey, and man, *Cancer Chemother Rep, 50*(4):219-244, 1966.

25. GEHAN, E. A.: A generalized Wilcoxon Test for comparing arbitrarily singly-censored samples, *Biometrika* (London), *52*:203-223, 1965.

26. GEHAN, E. A.: Some considerations in the planning of a clinical trial, *Proc of the VI International Biometric Conference*, Sydney, Australia, 1967.

27. GEHAN, E. A.: Estimating of survival functions from the life-table. *J Chronic Dis, 21*:629-44, 1969.

28. GEHAN, E. A., and THOMAS, D. G.: The performance of some two-sample tests in small samples with and without censoring, *Biometrika* (London), *56*:127-132, 1969.

29. GREENBERG, B. G.: Why randomize? *Biometrics, 7*:309, 1951.

30. GRIZZLE, J. E.: Multivariate comparison of results of treatment in chronic lympho-cytic and chronic granulocytic leukemia, *J Chronic Dis, 17*:127-152, 1964.

31. HILL, A. B.: *Statistical Methods in Clinical and Preventive Medicine.* Edinburgh and London, E. & S. Livingstone, 1962, pp. 610.

32. HOFFER, A.: A theoretical examination of double-blind design, *Canad Med Assn, 97*:123-127, 1967.

33. KAPLAN, E. L., and MEIER, P.: Non-parametric estimation from incomplete obser-vations, *J Amer Statis Assn, 53*(1):457-482, 1958.

34. LILIENFELD, A. M.: Emotional and other selected characteristics of cigarette smokers and nonsmokers as related to epidemiological studies of lung cancer and other diseases, *J Nat Cancer Inst, 22*(2):254-282, 1959.

35. LILIENFELD, A. M.; PEDERSON, E., and DOWD, J. E.: *Cancer Epidemiology: Methods of Study.* Baltimore, Johns Hopkins, 1967, pp. 165.

36. MANTEL, N.: Rapid estimation of standard errors of means for small samples, *Amer Statistician, 5*:26-27, October 1951.

37. MANTEL, N., and HAENSZEL, W.: Statistical aspects of the analysis of data from retrospective studies of disease, *J Nat Cancer Inst, 22*(4):719-748, 1959.

38. MANTEL, N.: Ranking procedures for arbitrarily restricted observation, *Biometrics, 23*(1):65-78, 1967.

39. MAXWELL, A. E.: *Analyzing Qualitative Data.* New York, Wiley, 1961, pp. 163.

40. PACKARD, F. R.: *The Life and Times of Ambrose Paré*, 2nd ed., New York, Hoeber, 1925, pp. 27, pp. 163.

41. PEARL, R.: Cancer and tuberculosis, *Amer J Hyg, 9*:97-159, 1929.

42. PLACKETT, R. L.: Current trends in statistical inference, *J Royal Statist Soc, 129* (2):249-267, 1966.

43. *Report of the Advisory Committee to the Surgeon General of the Public Health Service on Smoking and Health.* Public Health Service Publication No. 1103, Washington, D.C., U.S. Government Printing Office, 1964, pp. 387.

44. ROTH, J. G., and ELVIDGE, R.: Glioblastoma multiforme: Clinical survey, *J Neuro-surg, 17*:736-750, 1960.

45. SELAWRY, O. S., *et al.*: New treatment schedule with improved survival in child-hood leukemia, *J Amer Med Assn, 194*:75-81, 1965.

46. SNEDECOR, G. W., and COCHRAN, W. G.: *Statistical Methods*, 6th ed., Ames, Iowa State, 1967, pp. 593.
47. WIJSMAN, R. A.: Contributions to the study of the question of association of diseases, *Hum Biol*, *30*:219-236, 1958.
48. WILCOXON, F.: Individual comparisons by ranking methods. *Biometrics* (London), *1*:80-83, 1945.
49. WYNDER, E. L., and GRAHAM, E. A.: Tobacco smoking as a possible etiological factor in bronchogenic carcinoma: A study of 684 proved cases, *JAMA*, *143*: 329-336, 1950.

DEFINITION OF TERMS AND FORMULAE

Alternative hypothesis—see **Hypothesis**

Average value—see **Statistics**

Chi-square (x^2) **tests**—tests the hypothesis that there is no real difference in the proportion of individuals responding in two independent groups (prospective studies) or that there is no association between the possession of a characteristic and the occurrence of a disease (retrospective studies).[*] A chi-square test is also used in testing the hypothesis of no real difference in proportions in matched samples [†] or in proportions in two groups adjusting for differences in one factor such as age.[‡]

Formulae used for chi-square are:

Independent samples: Chi-square $= \dfrac{N(\mid ad - bc \mid - N/2)^2}{n_1 n_2 m_1 m_2}$

Matched samples: Chi-square $= (\mid g - h \mid - 1)^2 / (g + h)$

Test of Association
Adjusting for Differences
in One Subclassification: Chi-square $= \dfrac{(\mid \Sigma\, a_i - \Sigma\, E(a_i) \mid - 1/2)^2}{\Sigma\, V(a_i)}$

All with one degree of freedom.

Degrees of freedom—the number of independent observations involved in the calculation of a statistic. For example, the number of degrees of freedom in a standard deviation is the total number of observations (n) minus one, since the average value ($\bar{x}$) of the sample is a linear function calculated from the data.

Hypothesis—statement about a real difference in proportions or average values or some other functions of the observations among groups.

Null hypothesis—statement that there is no real difference in proportions or average values, etc. among groups.

Alternative hypothesis—statement that there is some real difference

---

[*] See appendix ii, 1.
[†] See appendix ii, 2.
[‡] See appendix ii, 3.

[50]

in proportions or average values, etc. among groups. A one-sided alternative specifies the direction of the real difference (either higher or lower) whereas a two-sided alternative specifies that the real difference may be in either direction.

Mean value—see average value under **Statistics**

Median value—see **Statistics**

Null hypothesis—see **Hypothesis**

One-sided test—see **Hypothesis**

Qualitative observations—see **Statistics**

Quantitative observations—see **Statistics**

Relative risk—the ratio of the proportion of individuals developing a disease among those having a characteristic to the proportion developing the disease among those not having the characteristic.*

Significance level—the probability of a difference in proportions, average values, etc. as great or greater than that observed arising by chance alone, assuming that the null hypothesis is true. When the probability is low and of the order of .05 or less, the null hypothesis is unlikely to be true.

Standard deviation—see **Statistics**

Standard error—see **Statistics**

Statistics—functions of a set of observations. Average (or mean) value, standard deviation, and standard error will be defined and formulae given for quantitative and qualitative observations.

A. *Quantitative observations*—a sample of n observations with measured values designated $x_1, x_2, \ldots, x_n$. The sample is assumed drawn randomly from a population of possible observations.

(1) *Average or mean* ($\bar{x}$)—is the sum of the sample observations divided by the number

$$\bar{x} = \frac{x_1 + x_2 + \ldots x_n}{n} = \frac{\sum\limits_{i=1}^{} x_i}{n}$$

where Σ means summation over the values of the subscript i and $i = 1, 2, \ldots, n$. The sample mean ($\bar{x}$) is an estimate of the true mean (μ) in the population.

---

* See appendix ii and iii for calculations related to formulae for measures of relative risk.

TABLE 17

TABLE OF χ^2

n.	P = .99.	.98.	.95.	.90.	.80.	.70.
1	.000157	.000628	.00393	.0158	.0642	.148
2	.0201	.0404	.103	.211	.446	.713
3	.115	.185	.352	.584	1.005	1.424
4	.297	.429	.711	1.064	1.649	2.195
5	.554	.752	1.145	1.610	2.343	3.000
6	.872	1.134	1.635	2.204	3.070	3.828
7	1.239	1.564	2.167	2.833	3.822	4.671
8	1.646	2.032	2.733	3.490	4.594	5.527
9	2.088	2.532	3.325	4.168	5.380	6.393
10	2.558	3.059	3.940	4.865	6.179	7.267
11	3.053	3.609	4.575	5.578	6.989	8.148
12	3.571	4.178	5.226	6.304	7.807	9.034
13	4.107	4.765	5.892	7.042	8.634	9.926
14	4.660	5.368	6.571	7.790	9.467	10.821
15	5.229	5.985	7.261	8.547	10.307	11.721
16	5.812	6.614	7.962	9.312	11.152	12.624
17	6.408	7.255	8.672	10.085	12.002	13.531
18	7.015	7.906	9.390	10.865	12.857	14.440
19	7.633	8.567	10.117	11.651	13.716	15.352
20	8.260	9.237	10.851	12.443	14.578	16.266
21	8.897	9.915	11.591	13.240	15.445	17.182
22	9.542	10.600	12.338	14.041	16.314	18.101
23	10.196	11.293	13.091	14.848	17.187	19.021
24	10.856	11.992	13.848	15.659	18.062	19.943
25	11.524	12.697	14.611	16.473	18.940	20.867
26	12.198	13.409	15.379	17.292	19.820	21.792
27	12.879	14.125	16.151	18.114	20.703	22.719
28	13.565	14.847	16.928	18.939	21.588	23.647
29	14.256	15.574	17.708	19.768	22.475	24.577
30	14.953	16.306	18.493	20.599	23.364	25.508

(2) *Median*—the value of the observation in the middle of the ordered sample of n observations. If n is an odd number, it is the value of the observation for the $(n+1)/2$ individual. When n is an even number, it is the average of the observations of the $(n/2)$ and $(n/2)+1$ individuals.

(3) *Standard deviation(s)*—a measure of variability of a single observation. It is the square root of the average of the squared deviations of each observation from the sample mean and has the same units as the original observations:

$$s = \sqrt{\frac{\sum_{i=1}^{n} (x_i - \bar{x})^2}{n - 1}}$$

or a formula that is simpler for purposes of calculation

$$s = \sqrt{\frac{n \sum_{i=1}^{n} x_i^2 - (\sum x_i)^2}{n(n - 1)}}$$

TABLE 17 (*Continued*)

.50.	.30.	.20.	.10.	.05.	.02.	.01.
.455	1.074	1.642	2.706	3.841	5.412	6.635
1.386	2.408	3.219	4.605	5.991	7.824	9.210
2.366	3.665	4.642	6.251	7.815	9.837	11.341
3.357	4.878	5.989	7.779	9.488	11.668	13.277
4.351	6.064	7.289	9.236	11.070	13.388	15.086
5.348	7.231	8.558	10.645	12.592	15.033	16.812
6.346	8.383	9.803	12.017	14.067	16.622	18.475
7.344	9.524	11.030	13.362	15.507	18.168	20.090
8.343	10.656	12.242	14.684	16.919	19.679	21.666
9.342	11.781	13.442	15.987	18.307	21.161	23.209
10.341	12.899	14.631	17.275	19.675	22.618	24.725
11.340	14.011	15.812	18.549	21.026	24.054	26.217
12.340	15.119	16.985	19.812	22.362	25.472	27.688
13.339	16.222	18.151	21.064	23.685	26.873	29.141
14.339	17.322	19.311	22.307	24.996	28.259	30.578
15.338	18.418	20.465	23.542	26.296	29.633	32.000
16.338	19.511	21.615	24.769	27.587	30.995	33.409
17.338	20.601	22.760	25.989	28.869	32.346	34.805
18.338	21.689	23.900	27.204	30.144	33.687	36.191
19.337	22.775	25.038	28.412	31.410	35.020	37.566
20.337	23.858	26.171	29.615	32.671	36.343	38.932
21.337	24.939	27.301	30.813	33.924	37.659	40.289
22.337	26.018	28.429	32.007	35.172	38.968	41.638
23.337	27.096	29.553	33.196	36.415	40.270	42.980
24.337	28.172	30.675	34.382	37.652	41.566	44.314
25.336	29.246	31.795	35.563	38.885	42.856	45.642
26.336	30.319	32.912	36.741	40.113	44.140	46.963
27.336	31.391	34.027	37.916	41.337	45.419	48.278
28.336	32.461	35.139	39.087	42.557	46.693	49.588
29.336	33.530	36.250	40.256	43.773	47.962	50.892

For larger values of n, the expression $\sqrt{2\chi^2} - \sqrt{2n-1}$ may be used as a normal deviate with unit variance.

The sample standard deviation is an estimate of the true standard deviation σ in the population. Variance is the square of a standard deviation and is designated s^2.

(4) *Standard error of sample mean* $s(\bar{x})$—measure of variability of a mean for n observations. The term standard error refers to measures of variability for functions of the observations such as standard error of the difference between means, ratio of two means, etc.

$$s(\bar{x}) = \frac{s}{\sqrt{n}}$$

Note that the standard error decreases directly in proportion to the square root of sample size. The interval $\bar{x} \pm 2s(\bar{x})$ is an approximate 95 per cent confidence interval for the true mean, that is, the true mean lies within the interval unless a random sample having 5 per cent chance is obtained. A confidence interval for the true mean of approximately 50 per cent is given by $\bar{x} \pm .6745\, s(\bar{x})$.

B. *Qualitative observations*–a sample of n observations which may take only values designated 0 or 1,* such as responder or non-responder, success or failure, etc. The sample is assumed to be drawn randomly from a population of observations. Formulae for qualitative observations yield exactly the same results that would be obtained by substitution of the values of 0 or 1 for each observation in the formulae for quantitative observations.

(1) *Proportion responding* $(\hat{p})$–the number of responders divided by the total number of observations. The sample proportion $\hat{p}$ is an estimate of the true proportion p in the population.

(2) *Standard error of proportion* $s(\hat{p})$–a measure of variability of a proportion based on n observations.

$$s(\hat{p}) = \sqrt{\frac{p(1-p)}{n}}$$

Note that the largest possible value for standard error is obtained when $p = .5$. Also, the standard error decreases in proportion to the square root of the number of observations.

Survival curve–the proportion of individuals surviving at a given time, $\hat{P}(t)$, plotted against time, t. The curve starts at 1.0 and decreases to zero when all individuals have died.

t-**test**–Student's test of the hypothesis that there is no real difference in average values in two groups of observations. The groups may be independent samples or paired samples.

Paired data:
$$t = \frac{\bar{d} - \delta}{s_d / \sqrt{n}}$$
with n − 1 degrees of freedom

Unpaired data:
$$t = \frac{\bar{x}_1 - \bar{x}_2 - (\mu_1 - \mu_2)}{s_p \sqrt{\frac{1}{n_1} + \frac{1}{n_2}}}$$
with $n_1 + n_2 - 2$ degrees of freedom

Test of hypothesis–rule for decision based on the value of some statistic, such as t or x^2 for deciding whether to accept a null hypothesis or reject it for an alternative hypothesis.

Two-sided test–see **Hypothesis**

---

* Qualitative observations may also refer to observations in several categories, such as 0—none, 1—mild, 2—moderate, 3—severe, etc. However, formulae given in this section are appropriate for data classified only into two categories.

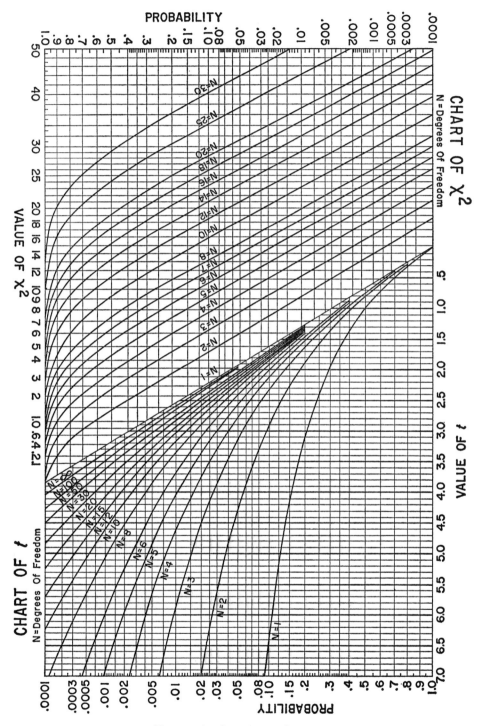

FIGURE 4. CHART OF χ^2 AND t

TABLE 18
TABLE OF t

n	P=.9	.8	.7	.6	.5	.4	.3	.2	.1	.05	.02	.01
1	.158	.325	.510	.727	1.000	1.376	1.963	3.078	6.314	12.706	31.821	63.657
2	.142	.289	.445	.617	.816	1.061	1.386	1.886	2.920	4.303	6.965	9.925
3	.137	.277	.424	.584	.765	.978	1.250	1.638	2.353	3.182	4.541	5.841
4	.134	.271	.414	.569	.741	.941	1.190	1.533	2.132	2.776	3.747	4.604
5	.132	.267	.408	.559	.727	.920	1.156	1.476	2.015	2.571	3.365	4.032
6	.131	.265	.404	.553	.718	.906	1.134	1.440	1.943	2.447	3.143	3.707
7	.130	.263	.402	.549	.711	.896	1.119	1.415	1.895	2.365	2.998	3.499
8	.130	.262	.399	.546	.706	.889	1.108	1.397	1.860	2.306	2.896	3.355
9	.129	.261	.398	.543	.703	.883	1.100	1.383	1.833	2.262	2.821	3.250
10	.129	.260	.397	.542	.700	.879	1.093	1.372	1.812	2.228	2.764	3.169
11	.129	.260	.396	.540	.697	.876	1.088	1.363	1.796	2.201	2.718	3.106
12	.128	.259	.395	.539	.695	.873	1.083	1.356	1.782	2.179	2.681	3.055
13	.128	.259	.394	.538	.694	.870	1.079	1.350	1.771	2.160	2.650	3.012
14	.128	.258	.393	.537	.692	.868	1.076	1.345	1.761	2.145	2.624	2.977
15	.128	.258	.393	.536	.691	.866	1.074	1.341	1.753	2.131	2.602	2.947
16	.128	.258	.392	.535	.690	.865	1.071	1.337	1.746	2.120	2.583	2.921
17	.128	.257	.392	.534	.689	.863	1.069	1.333	1.740	2.110	2.567	2.898
18	.127	.257	.392	.534	.688	.862	1.067	1.330	1.734	2.101	2.552	2.878
19	.127	.257	.391	.533	.688	.861	1.066	1.328	1.729	2.093	2.539	2.861
20	.127	.257	.391	.533	.687	.860	1.064	1.325	1.725	2.086	2.528	2.845
21	.127	.257	.391	.532	.686	.859	1.063	1.323	1.721	2.080	2.518	2.831
22	.127	.256	.390	.532	.686	.858	1.061	1.321	1.717	2.074	2.508	2.819
23	.127	.256	.390	.532	.685	.858	1.060	1.319	1.714	2.069	2.500	2.807
24	.127	.256	.390	.531	.685	.857	1.059	1.318	1.711	2.064	2.492	2.797
25	.127	.256	.390	.531	.684	.856	1.058	1.316	1.708	2.060	2.485	2.787
26	.127	.256	.390	.531	.684	.856	1.058	1.315	1.706	2.056	2.479	2.779
27	.127	.256	.389	.531	.684	.855	1.057	1.314	1.703	2.052	2.473	2.771
28	.127	.256	.389	.530	.683	.855	1.056	1.313	1.701	2.048	2.467	2.763
29	.127	.256	.389	.530	.683	.854	1.055	1.311	1.699	2.045	2.462	2.756
30	.127	.256	.389	.530	.683	.854	1.055	1.310	1.697	2.042	2.457	2.750
∞	.12566	.25335	.38532	.52440	.67449	.84162	1.03643	1.28155	1.64485	1.95996	2.32634	2.57582

Variance—see **Statistics**

Wilcoxon test (generalized)*—a test of the hypothesis that there is no real difference between two survival curves. The test is not dependent on any assumptions about the theoretical forms of the survival curves in the two groups.

---

* See appendix v, 2 for calculations and formulae.

CHI-SQUARE (X^2) TESTS OF ASSOCIATION OR DIFFERENCE IN PROPORTIONS

THE CHI-SQUARE TEST is used when the data to be analyzed are qualitative. Chi-square tests of association or difference in proportion are given for two independent samples, matched samples, and two independent samples adjusting for differences in one subclassification such as age.

(1) Independent Samples (2 X 2 Tables)

This test is used to test for an association between factors in retrospective studies of cases and their controls or to test the difference between proportions in retrospective or prospective studies. The appropriate tabular arrangement is given in the following table with the data from the study by Fisher *et al.*,[21] on response to mammary cancer to adjuvant Thio-TEPA.

TABLE 19
TABULAR ARRANGEMENT OF QUALITATIVE DATA FOR X^2 TEST

	Observed Data			
Category	With Characteristic or Successes	Without Characteristic or Failures	Total	Proportion with Characteristic or of Successes
Cases or Group 1	a = 15	b = 8	n_1 = 23	a/n_1 = .65
Controls or Group 2	c = 31	d = 5	n_2 = 36	c/n_2 = .86
	m_1 = 46	m_2 = 13	N = 59	m_1/N = .78

Where $N = a+b+c+d = n_1+n_2 = m_1+m_2$

Here, a, b, c, d are the numbers of observations in the four cells of the table and m_1, m_2 and n_1, n_2 are the numbers in the margins of the table. Thus, a is the number of cases with the characteristic or successes, etc.

According to the null hypothesis, either there is no association between possession of the characteristic and occurrence of the disease (retrospective studies) or there is no difference in the proportion of successes between the two groups (prospective or retrospective studies). If the null hypothesis is true, then the best estimate of the proportion with the characteristic or of successes is m_1/N = .78. Assuming this proportion of individuals possessed the characteristic (or succeeded) in each group, the following table can be constructed:

[58]

TABLE 20

EXPECTED DATA ASSUMING THE NULL HYPOTHESIS IS TRUE

Category	Expected Data		
	With Characteristic or Successes	*Without Characteristic or Failures*	*Total*
Cases or Group 1	$\dfrac{n_1\,m_1}{N} = 17.9$	$\dfrac{n_1\,m_2}{N} = 5.1$	$n_1 = 23$
Controls or Group 2	$\dfrac{n_2\,m_1}{N} = 28.1$	$\dfrac{n_2\,m_2}{N} = 7.9$	$n_2 = 36$
	$m_1 = 46$	$m_2 = 13$	$N = 59$

As an example, the expected number of cases with the characteristic is
23 (.78) $= 17.9$, since 78 per cent of the cases in each group are expected
to have the characteristic. The remaining three cells in the table can be
obtained by subtraction from the appropriate marginal totals or by the
formulae given above. The value of chi-square used in the test is

$$\text{Chi-square} = \text{Sum over all cells} \; \frac{(\,|\,\text{Observed} - \text{Expected}\,| - 1/2)^2}{\text{Expected}}$$

$$= \frac{(2.4)^2}{17.9} + \frac{(2.4)^2}{5.1} + \frac{(2.4)^2}{28.1} + \frac{(2.4)^2}{7.9} = 2.38$$

with one degree of freedom. In these calculations | Observed-Expected |
means absolute value, that is, the difference is always taken as positive.
Note that | Observed-Expected | is the same in all four cells of the 2 $\times$ 2
table; the value 1/2 is subtracted to improve the approximation in the
calculation of the probability of a chi-square value. There is one degree
of freedom because determining one expected value with the given set of
totals in the margins of the table is sufficient to determine all four expected
values by subtraction from the appropriate marginal total.

An abridged formula for chi-square is

$$\chi^2 = \frac{N\,(\,|\,ad - bc\,| - N/2)^2}{n_1\,n_2\,m_1\,m_2} = \frac{59\,(\,|\,(15)\,(5) - (8)\,(31)\,| - 59/2)^2}{(46)\,(13)\,(23)\,(36)} = 2.38$$

This formula is recommended when there are many values to calculate.
Otherwise the longer formula is preferred, since it shows the direction
and the magnitude of the difference between observed and expected values
in each cell. The calculated value of chi-square is then referred to tables
of the chi-square distribution with one degree of freedom to determine
the level of significance.

TABLE 21

VALUE OF CHI-SQUARE NECESSARY FOR SIGNIFICANCE AT GIVEN LEVEL
(TWO-SIDED TEST)

Degree of Freedom	20 Per Cent	10 Per Cent	5 Per Cent	1 Per Cent	.1 Per Cent
1	1.67	2.71	3.84	6.63	10.83

The value of chi-square obtained, 2.38, is about the 13 per cent level in the distribution (two-sided test). Consequently, the significance level of these data for a one-sided test is approximately 6 to 7 per cent, and these data provide suggestive evidence that the proportion with the characteristic is smaller in group 1 than group 2.

(2) Matched Samples (2 × 2 Tables)

The chi-square test for matched samples requires that individuals be classified according to the characteristics for which adjustments are made in the analysis such as age group, sex, severity of disease, etc. Patients are assigned to pairs so that each member of a pair has the same set of characteristics. The general arrangement for data from retrospective or prospective studies is given in the following table with data of Lilienfeld[34] to illustrate the calculations. The following possibilities exist for each pair of individuals in a prospective study, for example:

TABLE 22

POSSIBLE RELATIONSHIPS BETWEEN
PAIRS IN MATCHED SAMPLES

Group 1	Group 2
Success	Success
Failure	Failure
Success	Failure
Failure	Success

Each pair of individuals is classified according to these possibilities and the total number of pairs of each type are allocated to a table such as the following:

TABLE 23

ARRANGEMENT OF DATA FROM MATCHED SAMPLES
FOR CHI-SQUARE TEST

	Category	With Disease or Characteristic or in Group 1		
		High Level of Factor or Successes	Low Level of Factor or Failures	Total
Without Disease or Characteristic or in Group 2	High Level of Factor or Successes	$f = 30$	$g = 111$	$c = 141$
	Low Level of Factor or Failures	$h = 192$	$j = 570$	$d = 762$
	Total	$a = 222$	$b = 681$	$N = 903$

Tested is whether the level of the factor is associated with the possession of the characteristic or disease (retrospective and prospective studies) or whether the percentage of successes is the same in the two groups. If, for example, there is no real difference in the percentage of successes in the two groups, the same number of successes is expected in the two groups; that is, $a = (f + h) = 222$ is expected to equal $c = (f + g) = 141$ among the $N = 903$ pairs of individuals. This can occur only when $g = h$, and the statistical test is simply whether or not g differs significantly from 50 per cent of $(g + h)$. The chi-square test is calculated as follows:

$$\chi^2 = (|g-h| - 1)^2 / (g+h) = (|111-192| - 1)^2 / (303) = 21.1$$

with one degree of freedom. Referring to table 21, 21.1 is larger than 10.83, the value for chi-square at the significance level of .1 per cent. Values for P may be obtained easily from the graph (Fig. 4) also.

(3) Test of Association or Difference in Proportions.
Adjusting for Differences in One Subclassification

This test is used to test an association in retrospective studies or to test a difference in proportions in prospective studies. The general arrangement of data from the paper by Wynder and Graham [49] are given in Table 24.

The columns of the table are designated a, b, ... and (1), (2) ... in order to define the entries in the table and for use in later calculations. Thus, a_1 is the number of individuals with the disease and the characteristic in the first subclassification, etc.

Within the ith subclassification (age group), the approximate relative risk associated with the disease may be written $a_i d_i / b_i c_i$. To test whether or not possession of the characteristic is associated with developing the disease, the observed number of diseased persons having the characteristic, a_1 may be compared with the expected number assuming a relative risk of unity,

$$E(a_i) = n_{1i} \, m_{1i} / N_i \ .$$

For example, the relative risk in the first subclassification is

$$a_1 d_1 / b_1 c_1 = (13)(20)/(1)(126) = 2.06$$

The observed number of diseased persons is

$$a_1 = 13$$

and this may be compared with the expected number,

$$E(a_1) = n_{11} \, m_{11} / N_1 = (14)(139)/(160) = 12.162.$$

TABLE 24
ARRANGEMENT OF DATA TO TEST A DIFFERENCE IN PROPORTIONS *

Subclassification (Level)	With Disease or Group 1			Without Disease or Group 2			Both Groups Combined		
	With Char. or Success a (1)	Without Char. or Failure b (2)	Total n_1 (3)	With Char. or Success c (4)	Without Char. or Failure d (5)	Total n_2 (6)	With Char. or Success m_1 (7)	Without Char. or Failure m_2 (8)	Total N (9)
1	$a_1 = 13$	$b_1 = 1$	$n_{11} = 14$	$c_1 = 126$	$d_1 = 20$	$n_{21} = 146$	$m_{11} = 139$	$m_{21} = 21$	$N_1 = 160$
2	$a_2 = 105$	$b_2 = 0$	$n_{12} = 105$	$c_2 = 148$	$d_2 = 16$	$n_{22} = 164$	$m_{12} = 253$	$m_{22} = 16$	$N_2 = 269$
3	$a_3 = 254$	$b_3 = 4$	$n_{13} = 258$	$c_3 = 189$	$d_3 = 21$	$n_{23} = 210$	$m_{13} = 443$	$m_{23} = 25$	$N_3 = 468$
4	$a_4 = 185$	$b_4 = 2$	$n_{14} = 187$	$c_4 = 137$	$d_4 = 23$	$n_{24} = 160$	$m_{14} = 322$	$m_{24} = 25$	$N_4 = 347$
5	$a_5 = 40$	$b_5 = 1$	$n_{15} = 41$	$c_5 = 75$	$d_5 = 25$	$n_{25} = 100$	$m_{15} = 115$	$m_{25} = 26$	$N_5 = 141$
Total	597	8	605	675	105	780	1272	113	1385

* Data of Wynder and Graham.[49]

The difference between a_i and $E(a_i)$ can be tested relative to its variance $V(a_i)$ within each subclassification. When there is a consistent association over the various subclassifications between the disease and the study characteristic, an overall test of significance is given by summing the difference between the observed and expected values of a_i and relating this to its variance.

$$\chi^2 = \frac{(\mid \Sigma\, a_i - \Sigma\, E\,(a_i) \mid -1/2)^2}{\Sigma\, V\,(a_i)}$$

with one degree of freedom where

Σ means summation over subclassifications

$$E(a_i) = (n_{1i}\, m_{1i})/N_{1i}$$

and

$$V(a_i) = (n_{1i}\, n_{2i}\, m_{1i}\, m_{2i})/N_i^2\,(N_i-1)$$

All of the numbers needed for the formulae are given in the table above. The expected values and the variances can be calculated by adding several columns to the previous table (numbers in parenthesis refer to columns in the table).

TABLE 25

EXPECTED VALUES AND VARIANCES *

	a	E(a) (3) (7) ——— (9) (1)	E(d) (6) (8) ——— (9) (11)	V(a) (10) (11) ——— (9)−1.0 (12)
Age Group		(10)	(11)	(12)
30–39	13	12.162	19.162	1.4657
40–49	105	98.755	9.754	3.5942
50–59	254	244.218	11.218	5.8665
60–69	185	173.527	11.527	5.7811
70–79	40	33.439	18.439	4.4042
Total	597	562.101	70.101	21.1117

* Data of Wynder and Graham[49].

The calculation of $E(d_i)$ is needed for the calculation of $V(a_i)$. As a check on the calculations, note that $a_i - E(a_i) = \Sigma d_i - \Sigma E(d_i)$. In this case,

$$\Sigma\, a_i - \Sigma E(a_i) = 597 - 562.101 = 34.899$$

$$\Sigma d_i - \Sigma E(d_i) = 105 - 70.101 = 34.899$$

This difference is needed in the calculation of a summary relative risk and is denoted $Y = 34.899$.

Finally

$$\chi^2 = \frac{(\mid \Sigma a_i - \Sigma E(a_i) \mid -1/2)^2}{\Sigma V(a_i)} = \frac{(\mid 597 - 562.101 \mid -1/2)^2}{21.1117} = 56.04$$

with one degree of freedom. Referring to table 21, 56.04 is larger than the chi-square value of 10.83 at the .1 per cent level of significance. Hence, these data provide very strong evidence against the null hypothesis. Therefore, smoking is highly associated with the development of bronchogenic carcinoma after adjustment for the difference in age distributions for smokers and nonsmokers.

MEASURES OF RELATIVE RISK IN
RETROSPECTIVE STUDIES

A COMMON PROBLEM IN A RETROSPECTIVE STUDY is to estimate the proportion of individuals developing a disease among those having a characteristic relative to the proportion developing the disease among those not
having the characteristic. The ratio of the two proportions is the relative
risk.

(1) Studies in Cases and Controls *

Calculations are illustrated with data from the study of Doll and Hill [20]
on the relationship between bronchogenic carcinoma and smoking.

$$\text{Relative Risk} = \frac{a/(a+c)}{b/(b+d)} = \frac{a(b+d)}{b(a+c)}$$

When the data are subclassified, the above formula is appropriate within
each subclassification, and the subscript i should be added to each letter
designation for the relative risk in the ith subclassification.

In a retrospective study, a sample of cases (diseased persons) and
controls (persons without disease) is taken, and the relative frequencies
$a/(a+b)$ and $c/(c+d)$ give the proportions of persons with the characteristic. However, these are not the quantities needed for the relative-risk
formula. If the disease is of low incidence, a good approximation to the
relative risk may be obtained, since a and b will be small relative to c
and d, and therefore, $(b+d)/(a+c)$ may be estimated by d/c. The
formula for relative risk is then (approximately) ad/bc. These data are
available from a retrospective study. Using the data from the Doll-Hill
study, the estimate of relative risk is $(647)(27)/(622)(2) = 14.0$, indicating that the risk of bronchogenic carcinoma is 14 times as great for a
smoker than for a nonsmoker.

(2) Study of Matched Samples †

Several measures of relative risk are proposed by Mantel and Haens-

---

* The general arrangement for the 2 × 2 table is given in appendix ii, 1.

† The general arrangement of the data and the notation for the resulting 2 × 2 table is
given in appendix ii, 2. The calculations are illustrated using data from Lilienfeld.[34]

zel.[37] Their suggested compromise formula for overall relative risk is

$$R = h/g$$

The estimate of relative risk from Lilienfeld's data* is

$$R = h/g = 192/111 = 1.73$$

The relative risk is significantly greater than one (P<.001).**

(3) Studies of Cases and Controls Adjusting for Differences in One Factor†

Calculations for studies of cases and controls adjusting for differences in one factor are illustrated with data from Wynder and Graham.[49] Mantel and Haenszel[37] discuss measures of overall relative risk when data are subclassified according to age and studied at two levels of a characteristic, such as smoking and abstention. Different measures of overall relative risk result from differences in weighting relative risks within each subcategory. The relative risks for each age group follow:†

TABLE 26
RELATIVE RISKS †

Age Group	Relative Risk
30–39	2.062
40–49	. . . . . .*
50–59	7.057
60–69	15.542
70–79	13.331
Total	11.608

† Data of Wynder and Graham.[49]
* The relative risk is undefined, since no nonsmokers in the 40-49 age group developed bronchogenic carcinoma.

The relative risk in the total line is known as the crude relative risk because the separate subclassifications of the data are ignored when it is calculated. It is defined by the following formula:

$$\text{Crude relative risk} = (\Sigma a_i\ \Sigma d_i) / (\Sigma b_i\ \Sigma c_i)$$
$$= (597)(105) / (8)(675) = 11.608$$

Two summary measures of relative risk recommended by Mantel and Haenszel§ are

$$R = \Sigma(a_id_i/N_i) / \Sigma(b_ic_i/N_i)$$

* See page 16.
** The chi-square test of whether the risk differs significantly from unity is given in appendix ii, 2.
† The general tabular arrangement of these data is presented in appendix ii, 3.
‡ The notation and the data needed for this table are given in appendix ii, 3.
§ The notation and data are given in appendix ii, 3.

$$\text{and } R_1 = \frac{(\Sigma a_i)(\Sigma d_i)}{(\Sigma b_i)(\Sigma c_i)} \Bigg/ \frac{\Sigma E(a_i) \Sigma E(d_i)}{\Sigma E(b_i) \Sigma E(c_i)}$$

Each of these measures has the property of equalling unity only when $\Sigma a_i = \Sigma E(a_i)$. The chi-square value in the test given in Appendix ii, 3 is zero when the relative risks (R, R_1) are one. Since the value for chi-square will be large when the relative risks are large, chi-square tests whether the relative risks are significantly different from unity. The preferred measure of relative risk in Mantel and Haenszel[37] is R. The numerator of R_1 is the crude relative risk so that R_1 may be considered an adjusted crude relative risk.

The calculation of these measures of relative risk is accomplished by adding columns to the previous table published by Wynder and Graham.*

TABLE 27

CALCULATIONS * FOR DETERMINATION OF
RELATIVE RISK, $R = \Sigma(ad/N)/\Sigma(bc/N)$

Age Group	$\dfrac{ad}{N}$ $\dfrac{(1)\ (5)}{(9)}$	$\dfrac{bc}{N}$ $\dfrac{(2)\ (4)}{(9)}$
30-39	1.625	0.788
40-49	6.245	0.000
50-59	11.397	1.615
60-69	12.262	0.789
70-79	7.092	0.532
Total	38.622	3.724

* Data of Wynder and Graham.[49]

Derivative computations:

$$\Sigma E(b_i) = \Sigma b_i + Y = 8 + 34.899 = 42.899$$
$$\Sigma E(c_i) = \Sigma c_i + Y = 675 + 34.899 = 709.899$$

Hence, the two summary measures of relative risk are

$$R = (38.622)/(3.724) = 10.371$$

and
$$R_1 = 11.608 \Bigg/ \frac{(562.101)(70.101)}{(42.899)(709.899)} = 11.608/1.2939 = 8.971$$

The chi-square test† indicates that both of these risks are significantly greater than one $(P < .001)$.

---

* Given in appendix ii, 3.

† Appendix ii, 3.

Appendix iv

THE *t* TEST

Tests of the Difference Between Two Average Values

THE *t* TEST MAY BE USED TO EXAMINE the hypothesis that there is no real difference between two average values either in paired or unpaired data. It is assumed that the variability of the measurements is unknown in each group.

(1) Paired Data

One member of each pair receives each treatment according to a random allocation, pairing having been designed so that similar types of individuals are in each pair. Alternatively, each individual receives two treatments in random order so that the effects of treatments are compared for each patient.

The following data from Student's original paper [22] are of the latter type.

TABLE 28

ADDITIONAL HOURS OF SLEEP GAINED BY THE USE OF
TWO TYPES OF TREATMENT

Patient	Treatment A	Treatment B	Difference (B−A)
1	0.7	1.9	1.2
2	−1.6	0.8	2.4
3	−0.2	1.1	1.3
4	−1.2	0.1	1.3
5	−0.1	−0.1	0
6	3.4	4.4	1.0
7	3.7	5.5	1.8
8	0.8	1.6	0.8
9	0	4.6	4.6
10	2.0	3.4	1.4

The sample mean difference is

$$\bar{d} = \frac{1.2 + 2.4 + \ldots + 1.4}{10} = 1.58 \text{ hours sleep}$$

and the standard deviation of the differences is

$$s_d = \sqrt{\frac{n\Sigma d_i^2 - (\Sigma d)^2}{n(n-1)}}$$

[68]

where n = number of differences

  d_i = individual differences, i = 1, ... , n

  $\Sigma d_i^2 = d_1^2 + d_2^2 + \ldots + d_n^2$, i.e. the sum of squares of individual differences

  Σd = sum of differences

Then

$$s_d = \sqrt{\frac{10\,(38.58) - (15.8)^2}{90}} = 1.23 \text{ hours sleep}$$

The hypothesis to be tested is

Null hypothesis: True mean difference $\delta = 0$

Alternative hypothesis: $\delta \neq 0$

This is a two-sided test. For a one-sided test, the alternative hypothesis would be either $\delta < 0$ or $\delta > 0$.

The statistic for testing the null hypothesis is

$$t = \frac{\bar{d} - \delta}{s_d/\sqrt{n}} = \frac{1.58 - 0}{1.23/\sqrt{10}} = 4.06$$

with $n - 1 = 9$ degrees of freedom. To find the significance level attained by these data, the calculated value of t is referred to table 18 which records the distribution with 9 degrees of freedom.

degrees of freedom	$t_{.10}$	$t_{.05}$	$t_{.02}$	$t_{.01}$
9	1.833	2.262	2.821	3.250

In the table, t_p means that the probability of obtaining a value larger than $+ t_p$ or smaller than $- t_p$ is p. The $t_{.01}$ value is 3.250 and the calculated t value is 4.06. Hence, the probability is less than .01 for obtaining an average difference in the sample greater than 1.58 or less than -1.58. The graph (Fig. 4) is more flexible with greater number of degrees of freedom.

  These data are statistically significant at the 1 per cent level. Therefore, it is concluded that the two treatments differ in their sleep-producing qualities. The chance of error in this statement is less than 1 per cent. The estimate of the average difference in hours of sleep gained with treatment B compared to treatment A is 1.58 hours.

(2) Unpaired Data

  The problem here is to test the difference between the averages of two independent samples. The number of individuals in each sample need not be equal. This situation arises in clinical trials when average values of

some measurement have been calculated for individuals on the two regimens of treatment. The notation used follows:

Symbol	Meaning
$\bar{x}_i$	Sample average (or mean) value of measurement in group i, i = 1, 2
μ_i	True average value (unknown) of measurement in group i, i = 1, 2
s_i^2	Sample estimate of variability in group i, i = 1, 2 where

$$s_i^2 = \frac{n_i \Sigma_j x_{ij}^2 - (\Sigma_j x_{ij})^2}{n_i (n_i - 1)}$$

n_i	Number of individuals in the ith group, i = 1, 2
x_{ij}	Value of the measurement for the jth individual in the ith group, j = 1, . . . , n_i, i = 1, 2
s_p	Pooled estimate of standard deviation of measurements where

$$s_p = \sqrt{\frac{(n_1-1) s_1^2 + (n_2-1) s_2^2}{n_1 + n_2 - 2}}$$

The hypothesis to be tested is

$\quad\quad H_o \; : \; \mu_1 = \mu_2$ (True means are equal)

against either

$\quad\quad H_1 \; : \; \mu_1 \neq \mu_2$ (True means not equal, two-sided test)

$\quad\quad H_2 \; : \; \mu_1 > \mu_2$ (True mean for group 1 greater than that for group 2, one-sided test)

The assumption is made that the true variances in each group are the
same.

The statistic for testing the null hypothesis is

$$t = \frac{\bar{x}_1 - \bar{x}_2 - (\mu_1 - \mu_2)}{s_p \sqrt{\dfrac{1}{n_1} + \dfrac{1}{n_2}}}$$

and, if the null hypothesis is true, this follows Student's t distribution with
$n_1 + n_2 - 2$ degrees of freedom. A value of t is calculated from the data,
and the significance level achieved is determined by referring to the table
or graph of the t distribution (Table 18).

A test to determine whether the average age of patients managed by
each of two types of operation is the same in a clinical trial may be used

as an example. In a sense, this is a test of the randomization. The randomization of patients should insure that patients are comparable with respect to age, sex, and other factors possibly related to response to treatment.

In the example, suppose

Treatment 1	*Treatment 2*
$\bar{x}_1 = 58$ years	$\bar{x}_2 = 55$ years
$n_1 = 20$ patients	$n_2 = 18$ patients
$s_1^2 = 45$	$s_2^2 = 65$

and the hypothesis to be tested is

$$H_o \; : \; \mu_1 - \mu_2 = 0 \quad \text{(no difference in true average ages)}$$
$$H_1 \; : \; \mu_1 - \mu_2 \neq 0 \quad \text{(some difference in true average ages)}$$

To calculate t, first the pooled standard deviation is needed. This is

$$s_p = \sqrt{\frac{(19)\,(45) + (17)\,(65)}{20 + 18 - 2}} = 7.38$$

and the calculated value of t is

$$t = \frac{58 - 55 - 0}{7.38\sqrt{\dfrac{1}{20} + \dfrac{1}{18}}} = 1.25$$

with 36 degrees of freedom. Referring this to the tables of the t distribution, we find

degrees of freedom	$t_{.30}$	$t_{.20}$
30	1.055	1.310
∞	1.036	1.282

The table does not provide t values for 36 degrees of freedom; however, the probability can be estimated by using the tables for 30 and ∞ (infinite number) degrees of freedom. (The graph in Fig. 4 may be used for a more accurate determination.) The calculated value of t is between $t_{.30}$ and $t_{.20}$; hence the probability is greater than .20 of obtaining a t value of 1.25 or greater or -1.25 or less. Hence, these data provide no real evidence that the true average ages differed between the groups receiving each type of operation. The above test requires that the variability of the measurement is the same in both groups. When there is a real difference in the variation in the measurements, an alternative test must be used.*

---

* See Snedecor and Cochran [46] (p. 114) for a discussion of the problem.

CALCULATION OF SURVIVAL CURVES AND TEST OF THE DIFFERENCE BETWEEN TWO SURVIVAL CURVES

THE SURVIVAL TIME OF A PATIENT after operation or the time from operation to first recurrence of disease is often used in the evaluation of a surgical procedure. The method of Kaplan and Meier [33] for estimating survivorship function (or survival curve) and a generalized Wilcoxon test [25] for testing the difference between two survivorship functions may be used when censored data are present, that is, when some individuals are alive or free of disease at the time of analysis. Calculations are illustrated with data from a study of glioblastoma multiforme.

(1) Calculations of a Survival Curve *

The procedure of Kaplan and Meier [33] permits calculation of $\hat{P}(t)$, the estimated proportion of individuals surviving at time t. The n observed times to death or times to censoring are labeled and listed in order [†] of increasing magnitude so that $0 \leq t'_1 \leq t'_2 \ldots \leq t'_n$. The value used for the interval in censored observations is either the length of time from operation or the length of time free of disease, depending on the type of survival study undertaken.

$$\hat{P}(t) = \pi_r [(n-r) / (n-r+1)]$$

where r assumes those values for which $t'_r < t$ and for which t'_r measures a time to death. The estimate $\hat{P}(t)$ is calculated at every temporal point for a death. The values of t'_i ($i = 1, \ldots, 21$) from the study of glioblastoma multiforme follow with censored observations labeled as plus values:

t_1',	t_2',	t_3',	t_4',	t_5',	t_6',	t_7',	t_8',	t_9',	t_{10}',	t_{11}',
1,	2,	2,	2,	2+,	6,	8,	8,	9,	9+,	13,

t_{12}',	t_{13}',	t_{14}',	t_{15}',	t_{16}',	t_{17}',	t_{18}',	t_{19}',	t_{20}',	t_{21}',
13+,	16,	17,	22+,	25+,	29,	34,	36+,	43+,	45+

Using the formula

$$\hat{P}(t) = \pi_r [(n-r) / (n-r+1)]$$

---

* A computer program is available for calculating $\hat{P}(t)$, from E. A. Gehan.

† When ordering a censored survival time that is tied with a time to death, censored time is always considered as the larger; hence 2+ is larger than 2.

the following values are obtained:

t	$\hat{P}(t)$
1	$20/21 = .952381$
2	$\hat{P}(1)\ (19/20)\ (18/19)\ (17/18) = 17/21 = .809524$
6	$\hat{P}(2)\ (15/16) = .758676$
8	$\hat{P}(6)\ (14/15)\ (13/14) = .657519$
9	$\hat{P}(8)\ (12/13) = .606941$
13	$\hat{P}(9)\ (10/11) = .551765$
16	$\hat{P}(13)\ (8/9) = .490458$
17	$\hat{P}(16)\ (7/8) = .429151$
29	$\hat{P}(17)\ (4/5) = .343321$
34	$\hat{P}(29)\ (3/4) = .257491$

To illustrate details of calculation, $\hat{P}(13)$ will be considered. Following the formula directly,

$$\hat{P}(13) = \frac{(20)\ (19)\ (18)\ (17)\ (15)\ (14)\ (13)\ (12)\ (10),}{(21)\ (20)\ (19)\ (18)\ (16)\ (15)\ (14)\ (13)\ (11)}$$

but this can also be written as

$$\hat{P}(13) = \hat{P}\ (9)\ (10/11)$$

Thus, the values of $\hat{P}(t)$ are developed recursively from those previously calculated. The survival curves for experimental and control patients given in Fig. 3 were recorded by the Calcomp plotter, and the median and other percentiles of survival time may be read directly from the chart.

(2) Test of the Difference Between Two Survival Curves

A modification of the Wilcoxon test[25] is used to determine whether or not there is a real difference between two survival curves. It is appropriate whether or not censored observations are present; when no censored observations are present, the test reduces to the ordinary Wilcoxon test. The test is conditioned by the pattern of failure and censored observations, and tables of the normal distribution are used to determine the level of significance. The data for the patients with glioblastoma multiforme provide a good illustration of the method for calculating the W statistic required for the test. It is assumed that n_1, n_2 individuals are allocated randomly to treatments A and B, respectively, and the following are observed:

$$x'_1, \ldots, x'_{r_1} \qquad r_1 \text{ censored} \left. \rule{0pt}{24pt} \right\}$$
$$x_{r_1+1}, \ldots, x_{n_1} \qquad n_1 - r_1 \text{ failures}$$

Treatment A

$$y'_1, \ldots, y'_{r_2} \qquad r_2 \text{ censored}$$
$$\left.\begin{array}{c}\\ \\\end{array}\right\} \text{Treatment B}$$
$$y_{r_2+1}, \ldots, y_{n_2} \qquad n_2 - r_2 \text{ failures}$$

where x_i, y_j are times to failure and x'_i, y'_j are times to censoring measured from time of entry into study.

The statistic needed for the test (W) can be described as follows. Every observation in the A group is compared with every observation in the B group (a total of $n_1 \times n_2$ comparisons). If the observation in A is definitely larger than that in B, a plus one is scored, e.g. $(6, 2)$, $(9+, 7)$. If the observation in A is definitely smaller than that in B, a minus one is scored, e.g. $(8, 12)$, $(13, 22+)$. If the two observations are equal or a definite decision cannot be made, zero is scored, e.g. $(2, 2)$, $(2+, 5)$, $(9+, 11+)$, $(8, 7+)$. W is the sum of the scores over all $n_1 \times n_2$ comparisons.

More formally, the score for each comparison is defined by

$$U_{ij} = \begin{cases} -1 & x_i < y_j \text{ or } x_i \leq y'_j \\ 0 & x_i = y_j \text{ or } (x'_i, y'_j) \text{ or } x'_i \leq y_j \text{ or } y'_j < x_i \\ +1 & x_i > y_j \text{ or } x'_i \geq y_j \end{cases}$$

and the statistic $W = \Sigma_{i, j} U_{ij}$ where the sum extends over all $n_1 \times n_2$ comparisons. There will be a contribution to W for all comparisons of the two samples when both patients have died (i.e. all x_i, y_j comparisons, except for ties) and in all comparisons when a patient censored from observation has survived longer than one who has failed (i.e. when $x'_i \geq y_j$ or when $x_i \leq y'_j$).

If there are no censored observations or ties, W is much simpler to calculate:

$$W = n_2 (n_1 + n_2 + 1) - 2T'$$

where T' is the sum of the ranks of the second sample in the ordered combined sample. To determine the rank of an observation, both samples are combined and the observations ordered from smallest to largest. The ordered observations are labeled with the ranks, $1, 2 \ldots, n_1 + n_2$. T' is then the sum of the ranks of the observations in the second sample. Either sample can be considered as the second; it is easier to calculate T' if the smaller sample is called the second.

When there is no real difference between the survival distributions and the null hypothesis is true, then the true average value of W is zero. The extent to which W departs from zero is a measure of the difference between survival distributions.

In order to test the significance of a departure of W from zero, an estimate of the variability of W is needed. Mantel[38] gives a formula that is simple to calculate and describe without elaborate algebraic formulation.

Consider the two samples as being pooled into a single sample of $n_1 + n_2$ observations. Compare each observation with the remaining $n_1 + n_2 - 1$ observations. For the ith observation ($i = 1, \ldots, n_1 + n_2$), let U_i be the number of observations than which the ith is definitely greater minus the number than which it is definitely less. An observation is definitely greater (less) than another if the score for the comparison is $+1$ (-1). Scores of zero do not affect the calculation. For example, if the pool consists of observations 2, 3+, 4, 5+, 6, then U_i for the observation 4 is $1 - 2 = -1$, since 4 is definitely larger than one observation (2), definitely smaller than two observations (5+, 6), and cannot be ranked with respect to one observation (3+). The score for the latter comparison is zero.

The statistic W is now calculated as $W = \sum\limits_{i=1}^{n_1} U_i$ where summation is over the U_i of sample A only. The variance of W is given by

$$\text{Var (W)} = \frac{n_1 \, n_2}{(n_1 + n_2)(n_1 + n_2 - 1)} \left(\sum_{i=1}^{n_1+n_2} U_i^2 \right)$$

When there are no ties or censored observations, then the formula becomes

$$\text{Var (W)} = \frac{n_1 \, n_2}{3} (n_1 + n_2 + 1)$$

To test the null hypothesis (H_o) that two survival distributions are equivalent, the formula is

$$Z = \frac{W - O}{\sqrt{\text{Var (W)}}}$$

Under H_o, this follows (approximately) a normal distribution with mean zero and variance one. For the approximation to be reasonably good, the sample size should be at least ten in each group. Large values of Z such as those outside ± 2 should lead to the rejection of H_o.

Proceeding with the test for the data from the study of patients with glioblastoma multiforme, the first way of calculating W* is as follows: Taking the experimental group as group A, the first observation, 1 week, is larger than the first observation in the control group, 0 weeks, so $+1$ is scored. The observation, 1 week, is smaller than the remaining 14 observations in the control group; the score for these comparisons is -14. The

---

* A computer program for calculating the W test is available.[25] The number of observations in each group and the times to failure and censoring are needed for the program. The program calculates W, $\sqrt{\text{Var (W)}}$, Z, and the significance level of the value of W.

total score for this and the remaining observations in the experimental group follows.

TABLE 29

OBSERVATIONS IN EXPERIMENTAL GROUP (A)

Observations:	1	2	2	2	2+	6	8	8	9	9+	13
Score:	−13	−12	−12	−12	+2	−9	−6	−6	−6	+4	−3

Observations:	13+	16	17	22+	25+	29	34	36+	43+	45+
Score:	+5	−3	−3	+5	+5	−1	0	+5	+6	+6

The total of these scores is $W = -48$, indicating that the overall survival experience favors the control group. A positive value of W would indicate a survival experience favoring the experimental group.

The second way of calculating W is described by Mantel[38] and this also gives an estimate of Var (W). The formula for W is

$$W = \sum_{i=1}^{n_1} U_i$$

where $U_i = R_{1i} - R_{2i}$. The R_i are calculated by first ordering the observations in ascending order; both samples combined and each observation labeled according to group. The following steps are executed:

TABLE 30

METHOD FOR CALCULATING W

Computation of R_1	*Computation of R_2*
Step 1: Rank from left to right omitting censored values.	*Step 4:* Rank from right to left including censored values.
Step 2: Assign next higher rank to censored values.	*Step 5:* Reduce the rank of tied observations to the lowest rank for the value.
Step 3: Reduce the rank of tied observations to the lowest rank for the value.	*Step 6:* Reduce the rank of censored observation to unity.

For actual data under consideration, the values are

Label:		A	A	A	A		A		A		A	A	A	A			A
Observations in ascending order:	0	1	2	2	2	2	2+ 5	6	7	7+ 8	8	9	9+ 11+	12	13		

R_{1i} { Step 1 / Step 2 / Step 3 }

Step 1: 1 2 3̸ 4̸ 5̸ 4̸   7 8 9   1̸0̸ 1̸1̸ 12   13 14
Step 2:   7   10   13 13
Step 3:   3 3 3 3   10 10

R_{2i} { Step 4 / Step 5 / Step 6 }

Step 4: 36 35 3̸4̸ 3̸3̸ 3̸2̸ 3̸1̸ 3̸0̸ 29 28 27 2̸6̸ 2̸6̸ 2̸4̸ 23 2̸2̸ 2̸1̸ 20 19
Step 5:   31 31 31 31   24 24
Step 6:   1   1   1 1

Compute

$U_i = R_{1i} - R_{2i}$ −35 −33 −28 −28 −28 −28 6 −22 −20 −18   9 −14 −14 −11 12 12 −7 −5

Label:	A	A	A		A		A	A		A		A		A	A		
Observations in ascending order (continued)	13+	16	17	19+22+22+25+29	30+34	35+36+39+42	43+45+	46	54

R_{1i} { Step 1 / Step 2 / Step 3 }

Step 1:   15 16   17   18   19   20 21
Step 2: 15   17 17 17 17   18   19 19 19   20 20
Step 3:

R_{2i} { Step 4 / Step 5 / Step 6 }

Step 4: 1̸8̸ 17 16 1̸6̸ 1̸4̸ 1̸6̸ 1̸2̸ 11 1̸0̸ 9 8̸ 7̸ 6̸ 5 4̸ 3̸ 2 1
Step 5:
Step 6: 1   1 1 1 1   1   1 1 1   1 1

Compute

$U_i = R_{1i} - R_{2i}$ 14 −2 0 16 16 16   6 17   9 18 18 18 14 19 19   18 20

The value of W is −33 −28 −28. . . +19 = −183 + 135 = −48, as before

The variance of W is

$$\text{Var (W)} = \frac{(21)\ (15)\ (11{,}894)}{(36)\ (35)} = 2973.5.$$

Then

$$\sqrt{\text{Var (W)}} = 54.53$$

and the test statistic is

$$Z = \frac{W - O}{\sqrt{\text{Var (W)}}} = \frac{-48}{54.53} < 1.$$

The value of Z is referred to tables of the normal distribution to calculate the probability of such a value of Z or greater. The values of Z, always taken as positive, to achieve significance at given levels are as follows:

TABLE 31

SIGNIFICANCE LEVEL RELATED TO VALUE OF Z

Two-sided Test	.60	.50	.40	.30	.20	.10	.050	.02	.010
One-sided Test	.30	.25	.20	.15	.10	.05	.025	.01	.005
Value of Z	.52	.67	.84	1.04	1.28	1.64	1.96	2.33	2.58

In the example, the hypotheses are:

H_o: No difference in survival curves between experimental and control.
H_1: Difference in survival curves favoring experimental group.

The calculated value of W is negative as is the value of Z. Hence, these data provide no real evidence that the over-all survival experience is better in the experimental group. To achieve a result significant at the .05 level, a positive value of W must be obtained along with a value of Z greater than +1.64. When there are censored observations in the two groups being compared, the W test is a relatively powerful evaluation of the difference between survival curves.[28]

RANDOMIZATION IN CLINICAL TRIALS

IN A COMPARATIVE (or Phase-III) trial, it is often desirable to assign the treatments to patients being entered into study in random order.[29] An essential feature of randomization procedure is that it should be objective and impersonal; it does not mean arranging treatments in some order that appears haphazard. There are several informal techniques for randomizing patients into groups for treatment such as flipping a coin, shuffling numbered cards, assigning patients with odd hospital numbers to one treatment and those with even numbers to another treatment, assigning patients according to the day of entry into the study or date of birth of the patient, etc. These methods often are applied to small studies, but the method for randomization usually selected is the use of tables of random numbers.

Procedures for randomization are usually carried out using cards with the names of the treatments in sealed envelopes numbered serially. When a patient is entered, the investigator opens an envelope according to the numbered order and administers the treatment named on the enclosed card. If the clinical trial is a cooperative venture involving several institutions, sets of numbered cards should be available at each institution. Alternatively, a system of entry of patients by telephone may be used. A call is placed by the investigator to the central office in which the randomization list is located. The latter technique is expensive but may be desirable for studies involving relatively small numbers of patients or when it is important for the central office to be completely informed about the entry of patients into study.

Separate randomizations are usually produced for major categories of disease such as stage of disease, severity of disease, diagnosis, etc. The number of categories should be limited to about four or less; otherwise each category will contain too few patients. Separate randomizations according to category of disease insure a balanced allocation of patients to treatments within all relevant subcategories.

Tables of random digits or random permutations are usual references for randomization procedures. A table of random digits such as table 34 is a series of digits $0\ldots\ldots9$ in which each digit occurs with approximately equal frequency and in which there is no systematic pattern. In a clinical trial comparing two treatments, a specific number of patients is chosen after which there will be an equal number of patients on the two programs of therapy. This restriction averts the possibility that a long sequence of patients will be assigned to either treatment. For two treatments, it is reasonable to require balance after four patients, assigning two to each treatment. The possible orders for assignments of two treatments A and B to four patients are

1. A B B A	4. B A B A
2. A B A B	5. A A B B
3. B A A B	6. B B A A

Since orders 5 and 6 may not seem random, although either is as likely as any other possible order, systematic orders such as 5 and 6 usually are eliminated from the possibilities. For a randomization list of twenty patients involving two treatments a method as convenient as any is to assign treatment orders to random digits in the following way.

TABLE 32

ASSIGNMENT OF ORDER OF TREATMENT
TO RANDOM DIGITS

Random Digits	Order of Treatments
00-24	A B B A
25-49	A B A B
50-74	B A A B
75-99	B A B A

A starting point is selected haphazardly in the table of random digits and the first five pairs of digits are recorded as they occur in the table proceeding in any direction from the starting point. Suppose the choices are 05, 35, 28, 49, 88. The first four patients receive treatments in order A B B A, the next four A B A B, the next four A B A B, and the last four patients receive B A B A. It is a simple matter to produce a long list of random assignments in this way.

For three or more treatments, one way to proceed would be to record treatments and random digits as follows:

Treatments: A, B, C, D, . . .

Random Digits: 0, 1, 2, 3, . . .

The restriction of the randomization would be decided, e.g. with three treatments no treatment should appear more than twice among the first six patients, with four treatments no treatment should appear more than twice among eight patients, etc. A series of single random digits could then be chosen from the table, in which all numbers other than those designating treatments would be rejected. For example, with four treatments, the sequence of numbers 1 3 2 3 0 0 5 2 1, leads to the assignment

B D C D A A C B. If any number appeared more than twice in the first eight patients, those times it appeared above two would be rejected by the restriction requirement. Unsatisfactory arrangements such as A A B B C C D D would be eliminated arbitrarily. The same type of technique could be used for a larger number of treatments.

The randomization technique described here is known as restricted randomization. The effect of such a procedure upon tests of significance has not been investigated fully but is almost certainly negligible. It has the advantage of producing balanced assignments of treatments to patients without the appearance of any systematic arrangements.

Planning and Analysis of Clinical Studies

TABLE 33
RANDOM DIGITS

23 64 18 82 84	97 06 93 64 24	86 16 32 47 50	79 01 90 73 17	15 43 16 74 99	81 28 04 56 64	61 51 25 43 32
46 59 62 33 62	90 08 34 76 99	34 10 27 00 32	36 65 69 33 60	95 13 54 19 49	63 24 64 53 61	23 50 12 29 68
22 17 50 89 46	83 67 07 06 71	87 39 66 36 63	55 93 24 79 24	50 84 40 23 16	26 93 46 19 98	69 18 33 16 16
15 02 56 35 92	91 46 90 79 22	00 21 71 37 56	46 11 15 63 44	89 50 55 12 04	53 90 40 79 79	14 03 45 16 54
62 94 56 20 94	21 73 25 53 59	74 02 64 48 96	78 48 37 56 72	28 02 22 33 62	42 20 10 44 35	85 65 57 64 39
61 82 00 65 62	38 92 74 75 43	85 55 52 88 25	64 81 48 74 12	60 19 84 01 64	08 80 44 87 61	36 73 04 19 89
34 65 95 68 15	21 04 05 63 29	27 81 13 36 24	75 31 85 87 54	33 73 78 22 94	19 11 64 70 48	66 03 18 51 70
52 43 85 30 58	94 19 20 85 97	78 99 63 63 02	00 04 91 77 11	35 48 07 17 33	27 82 59 27 20	65 52 54 85 78
78 34 19 75 71	71 65 71 09 85	61 30 29 54 72	09 10 34 89 50	06 68 13 89 40	26 32 96 31 68	20 01 07 52 26
77 77 27 51 90	06 13 83 02 28	47 56 20 26 46	08 56 32 31 10	41 68 46 33 69	13 10 53 86 94	25 56 88 68 39
28 40 86 66 46	64 47 82 84 01	70 92 02 46 39	99 63 42 70 20	06 16 37 82 26	44 91 32 27 88	90 97 93 79 75
29 27 96 31 77	69 21 07 15 04	32 23 64 77 03	44 98 99 29 79	43 95 17 58 61	97 27 11 13 82	54 03 56 13 02
10 35 65 10 12	72 90 95 01 87	16 10 84 29 12	67 11 61 83 72	82 84 58 15 45	31 76 73 28 35	88 37 49 20 33
40 32 34 65 99	06 45 96 83 67	91 79 56 00 57	94 68 20 58 09	50 42 52 86 92	13 40 69 75 77	10 25 85 25 01
59 48 42 06 18	08 49 26 41 75	62 96 81 28 41	41 86 28 36 89	46 95 36 33 76	76 99 28 74 89	37 49 00 71 82
79 57 73 33 02	55 70 55 85 32	19 60 23 35 00	63 66 04 68 76	22 17 75 33 58	15 41 30 04 69	82 24 78 51 18
80 58 40 78 63	43 16 62 18 16	61 82 97 47 25	95 80 40 33 69	36 19 19 04 06	93 05 23 20 05	61 87 11 59 38
83 65 43 96 06	25 68 42 65 39	56 73 31 37 87	42 01 18 81 78	76 98 59 39 18	68 99 30 77 48	56 57 59 82 78
09 44 31 28 60	68 90 22 71 12	13 93 21 30 54	79 13 10 78 88	02 13 92 55 40	85 62 56 37 86	71 66 07 08 05
16 88 58 18 93	41 54 63 27 26	18 34 95 37 16	50 23 96 92 17	99 74 78 71 35	79 40 99 12 35	73 69 29 87 76
52 49 44 41 15	19 45 73 57 61	92 11 69 59 21	62 09 89 79 99	20 75 96 44 36	69 20 63 52 29	39 21 41 70 06
00 28 35 39 59	73 16 14 00 05	31 42 09 28 73	81 88 67 61 00	34 24 81 04 35	52 63 29 29 11	06 24 34 39 07
23 35 85 55 14	73 36 64 94 93	55 79 48 33 04	62 90 85 18 30	74 64 20 88 01	07 74 80 22 57	16 43 47 46 43
13 05 82 65 05	82 60 15 61 17	55 31 77 62 44	81 30 28 67 19	44 00 77 74 72	16 76 47 99 33	00 34 88 45 49

TABLE 33 (Continued)

23	91	91	23	71	62	73	30	17	71	92	23	59	80	34	22	40	18	62	93	89	41	51	78
61	24	10	03	60	39	25	50	97	07	68	26	50	96	75	15	32	92	58	48	44	10	47	44
36	51	66	93	03	91	97	14	77	52	29	09	02	61	10	89	71	87	02	96	39	71	80	71
75	19	54	97	37	57	48	22	32	38	68	48	59	14	63	98	54	10	98	54	48	34	25	45
68	62	28	41	89	05	16	58	21	38	06	18	93	97	81	07	71	39	84	05	94	01	00	55
87	02	04	71	61	27	72	04	87	96	67	95	61	76	18	96	45	14	59	32	70	34	17	25
54	34	07	04	26	17	48	23	44	69	85	31	21	55	37	89	66	58	58	13	63	20	72	88
19	99	55	58	05	39	57	80	83	44	83	00	16	17	02	19	09	51	97	91	06	67	79	21
76	87	39	64	04	85	72	44	54	63	81	49	74	24	82	98	45	66	34	42	81	37	07	52
94	00	76	57	01	56	18	78	61	56	85	91	09	49	68	66	92	33	97	96	54	32	38	43
97	68	26	20	38	31	11	64	43	78	77	25	68	10	84	01	89	32	15	62	75	37	94	56
31	19	39	62	33	02	52	96	84	02	48	94	37	93	57	69	52	06	33	92	18	72	99	78
76	02	63	87	04	41	74	17	17	43	72	89	11	24	25	01	77	93	82	47	43	49	89	56
37	81	31	45	08	49	54	88	60	21	82	90	95	53	24	81	10	15	30	98	92	54	08	04
58	92	77	69	35	85	76	30	60	01	41	43	78	51	62	13	64	08	79	13	14	24	82	98
46	86	72	41	68	21	15	61	24	75	07	77	04	77	72	33	71	51	81	04	98	65	74	33
12	24	99	66	32	55	96	47	04	97	97	31	01	99	20	79	41	31	79	33	32	07	88	02
80	60	76	05	62	92	82	01	45	70	42	67	71	06	91	29	66	25	26	24	27	32	79	55
33	53	68	03	22	96	66	10	52	55	50	01	25	47	51	34	59	09	82	47	56	26	37	28
81	18	87	54	55	59	90	57	07	07	19	79	77	31	11	84	16	84	00	33	16	69	12	79
63	11	00	42	77	79	55	54	65	22	40	80	42	97	69	71	46	13	00	91	79	73	17	88
12	90	25	52	66	48	64	43	53	16	79	86	40	71	99	00	53	28	47	77	05	85	99	04
87	20	51	64	36	95	64	57	67	57	48	16	34	52	87	55	39	66	86	49	86	84	72	19
68	35	18	12	27	03	25	38	23	92	52	65	14	99	49	17	90	88	53	45	31	56	76	96
06	32	66	13	53	27	70	58	63	86	79	81	40	42	75	55	90	31	29	98	85	32	41	42
89	87	33	00	93	01	52	62	96	13	95	14	99	97	37	19	04	07	85	30	21	92	62	87
67	22	71	13	99	16	13	50	17	84	99	03	49	11	07	09	43	69	55	29	76	39	29	20
58	61	75	22	55	70	76	40	28	39	55	75	44	82	76	43	97	82	96	23	60	44	21	68
07	01	31	64	15	19	89	89	66	91	84	47	80	30	48	39	15	52	48	14	73	26	92	91
39	38	64	63	22	69	90	39	38	58	96	52	09	09	40	33	20	69	70	52	98	63	86	08
30	66	17	14	33	99	92	47	56	75	99	09	29	99	34	61	62	16	38	18	46	75	72	62
19	02	74	35	49	73	26	40	88	46	78	07	73	06	87	13	88	25	33	99	15	40	47	78
99	49	87	90	19	94	29	28	72	07	43	35	94	05	71	25	45	34	98	22	51	66	96	69
58	93	23	31	48	73	85	60	13	77	77	08	51	76	46	18	45	85	72	84	33	26	53	24
14	00	04	32	96	22	16	10	85	05	44	12	86	37	21	48	99	94	62	07	76	21	67	79

INFORMED CONSENT

THE CONDUCT OF CLINICAL TRIALS raises moral and ethical as well as scientific questions. Essential to any such investigation is informed consent of the patient or volunteer. The investigator is obligated to divulge full information about the trial to those entering it or to those responsible in the case of minors. A form for consent to be signed by the patient on a voluntary basis, which has been found useful, appears in Figure 5. The Nuremberg code and events leading to it have elicited protracted discussions. The following excerpt from the code gives the flavor of its admonitions.

Rule 1. "The voluntary consent of the human subject is absolutely essential. . . . The duty and responsibility for ascertaining the quality of consent rests upon each individual who initiates, directs, or engages in the experiment. It is a personal duty and responsibility which may not be delegated to another with impunity.

Rule 2. "The experiment should be such as to yield fruitful results for the good of society unprocurable by other methods or means of study, and not random or unnecessary in nature.

Rule 3. "The experiment should be so designed and based on the results of animal experimentation and a knowledge of the natural history of the disease or other problem under study that the anticipated results will justify the performance of the experiment.

Rule 4. "The experiment should be so conducted as to avoid all unnecessary physical and mental suffering and injury.

Rule 5. "No experiment should be conducted wherein there is an *a priori* reason to believe that death or disabling injury will occur; except, perhaps, in those experiments where the experimental physicians also serve as subjects.

Rule 6. "The degree of risk to be taken should never exceed that determined by the humanitarian importance of the problem to be solved by the experiment."

The code has been criticized because of certain ambiguities. For example, the implication in Rule 2 that the end might justify the means for the good of society has received its share of adverse comment. Also, the latter part of Rule 5 is a statement alien to the precepts of morality in the view of some readers.

The principles of medical ethics of the American Medical Association require adherence to the following rules:

THE UNIVERSITY OF TEXAS
M. D. ANDERSON HOSPITAL AND TUMOR INSTITUTE

CONSENT TO INVESTIGATIONAL
PROCEDURE OR TREATMENT

PATIENT_____ UNIT NO. _____

1. I HEREBY AUTHORIZE DR. _____, THE ATTENDING PHYSICIAN, AND/OR
    THE PHYSICIAN HE MAY DESIGNATE TO PERFORM THE FOLLOWING PROCEDURE OR TREATMENT:

    _____

    _____

    _____ ON _____
                                                      NAME OF PATIENT OR MYSELF

2. THE NATURE AND PURPOSE OF THE PROCEDURE OR TREATMENT, POSSIBLE ALTERNATIVE METHODS OF
    TREATMENT, THE RISKS INVOLVED AND THE POSSIBILITY OF COMPLICATIONS HAVE BEEN EXPLAINED TO
    ME BY DR. _____. I FULLY UNDERSTAND THAT THE PROCEDURE OR
    TREATMENT TO BE PERFORMED IS INVESTIGATIONAL, THAT IT MAY INVOLVE MORE THAN ORDINARY RISK,
    AND IS UNPROVED BY MEDICAL EXPERIENCE. WITH FULL KNOWLEDGE OF THIS, I VOLUNTARILY CONSENT
    TO THE PROCEDURE OR TREATMENT DESIGNATED IN PARAGRAPH 1 ABOVE UPON _____

    _____.
    NAME OF PATIENT OR MYSELF

    _____   _____
                 DATE   TIME

    WITNESS:_____   SIGNED:_____
                 ATTENDING PHYSICIAN   PATIENT OR PERSON RESPONSIBLE

    WITNESS:_____   _____
                                                            RELATIONSHIP

    VERIFICATION OF EXPLANATION AND PATIENT CONSENT SHOULD BE RECORDED IN THE PROGRESS
    NOTES OF THE MEDICAL RECORD.

FIGURE 5. FORM FOR INFORMED CONSENT

1. "The voluntary consent of the person on whom the experiment is to be performed must be obtained.

2. "The danger of each experiment must have been investigated previously by means of animal experimentation.

3. "The experiment must be performed under proper medical protection and management."

The central objective of all codifications is usually the protection of the rights of the individual. In no activity of the medical profession is the delicate balance with public opinion and legal restriction more delicate than in the comparative clinical trial. The investigator who proposes a clinical trial must carefully weigh the manner in which he is discharging this responsibility, since no set of rules is likely to cover every situation encountered in the course of such experimentation.

---

* Tables beginning on pages 92 and 93 are taken from *Experimental Designs*[13] by W. G. Cochran and G. M. Cox and the multiplier table on page 94 from *Statistical Methods*[46] by G. W. Snedecor and W. G. Cochran and the chart was redrawn from an original by J. F. Crow.[17] Tables of χ^2 and t are taken from Fisher: *Statistical Methods for Research Workers*[22] published by Oliver & Boyd, Ltd., Edinburgh, and by permission of the author and publishers.

TABLE OF χ^2

n.	P = .99.	.98.	.95.	.90.	.80.	.70.
1	.000157	.000628	.00393	.0158	.0642	.148
2	.0201	.0404	.103	.211	.446	.713
3	.115	.185	.352	.584	1.005	1.424
4	.297	.429	.711	1.064	1.649	2.195
5	.554	.752	1.145	1.610	2.343	3.000
6	.872	1.134	1.635	2.204	3.070	3.828
7	1.239	1.564	2.167	2.833	3.822	4.671
8	1.646	2.032	2.733	3.490	4.594	5.527
9	2.088	2.532	3.325	4.168	5.380	6.393
10	2.558	3.059	3.940	4.865	6.179	7.267
11	3.053	3.609	4.575	5.578	6.989	8.148
12	3.571	4.178	5.226	6.304	7.807	9.034
13	4.107	4.765	5.892	7.042	8.634	9.926
14	4.660	5.368	6.571	7.790	9.467	10.821
15	5.229	5.985	7.261	8.547	10.307	11.721
16	5.812	6.614	7.962	9.312	11.152	12.624
17	6.408	7.255	8.672	10.085	12.002	13.531
18	7.015	7.906	9.390	10.865	12.857	14.440
19	7.633	8.567	10.117	11.651	13.716	15.352
20	8.260	9.237	10.851	12.443	14.578	16.266
21	8.897	9.915	11.591	13.240	15.445	17.182
22	9.542	10.600	12.338	14.041	16.314	18.101
23	10.196	11.293	13.091	14.848	17.187	19.021
24	10.856	11.992	13.848	15.659	18.062	19.943
25	11.524	12.697	14.611	16.473	18.940	20.867
26	12.198	13.409	15.379	17.292	19.820	21.792
27	12.879	14.125	16.151	18.114	20.703	22.719
28	13.565	14.847	16.928	18.939	21.588	23.647
29	14.256	15.574	17.708	19.768	22.475	24.577
30	14.953	16.306	18.493	20.599	23.364	25.508

TABLE OF χ^2 (*Continued*)

.50.	.30.	.20.	.10.	.05.	.02.	.01.
.455	1.074	1.642	2.706	3.841	5.412	6.635
1.386	2.408	3.219	4.605	5.991	7.824	9.210
2.366	3.665	4.642	6.251	7.815	9.837	11.341
3.357	4.878	5.989	7.779	9.488	11.668	13.277
4.351	6.064	7.289	9.236	11.070	13.388	15.086
5.348	7.231	8.558	10.645	12.592	15.033	16.812
6.346	8.383	9.803	12.017	14.067	16.622	18.475
7.344	9.524	11.030	13.362	15.507	18.168	20.090
8.343	10.656	12.242	14.684	16.919	19.679	21.666
9.342	11.781	13.442	15.987	18.307	21.161	23.209
10.341	12.899	14.631	17.275	19.675	22.618	24.725
11.340	14.011	15.812	18.549	21.026	24.054	26.217
12.340	15.119	16.985	19.812	22.362	25.472	27.688
13.339	16.222	18.151	21.064	23.685	26.873	29.141
14.339	17.322	19.311	22.307	24.996	28.259	30.578
15.338	18.418	20.465	23.542	26.296	29.633	32.000
16.338	19.511	21.615	24.769	27.587	30.995	33.409
17.338	20.601	22.760	25.989	28.869	32.346	34.805
18.338	21.689	23.900	27.204	30.144	33.687	36.191
19.337	22.775	25.038	28.412	31.410	35.020	37.566
20.337	23.858	26.171	29.615	32.671	36.343	38.932
21.337	24.939	27.301	30.813	33.924	37.659	40.289
22.337	26.018	28.429	32.007	35.172	38.968	41.638
23.337	27.096	29.553	33.196	36.415	40.270	42.980
24.337	28.172	30.675	34.382	37.652	41.566	44.314
25.336	29.246	31.795	35.563	38.885	42.856	45.642
26.336	30.319	32.912	36.741	40.113	44.140	46.963
27.336	31.391	34.027	37.916	41.337	45.419	48.278
28.336	32.461	35.139	39.087	42.557	46.693	49.588
29.336	33.530	36.250	40.256	43.773	47.962	50.892

For larger values of n, the expression $\sqrt{2\chi^2} - \sqrt{2n-1}$ may be used as a normal deviate with unit variance.

TABLE OF *t*

n	P = .9	.8	.7	.6	.5	.4	.3	.2	.1	.05	.02	.01
1	.158	.325	.510	.727	1.000	1.376	1.963	3.078	6.314	12.706	31.821	63.657
2	.142	.289	.445	.617	.816	1.061	1.386	1.886	2.920	4.303	6.965	9.925
3	.137	.277	.424	.584	.765	.978	1.250	1.638	2.353	3.182	4.541	5.841
4	.134	.271	.414	.569	.741	.941	1.190	1.533	2.132	2.776	3.747	4.604
5	.132	.267	.408	.559	.727	.920	1.156	1.476	2.015	2.571	3.365	4.032
6	.131	.265	.404	.553	.718	.906	1.134	1.440	1.943	2.447	3.143	3.707
7	.130	.263	.402	.549	.711	.896	1.119	1.415	1.895	2.365	2.998	3.499
8	.130	.262	.399	.546	.706	.889	1.108	1.397	1.860	2.306	2.896	3.355
9	.129	.261	.398	.543	.703	.883	1.100	1.383	1.833	2.262	2.821	3.250
10	.129	.260	.397	.542	.700	.879	1.093	1.372	1.812	2.228	2.764	3.169
11	.129	.260	.396	.540	.697	.876	1.088	1.363	1.796	2.201	2.718	3.106
12	.128	.259	.395	.539	.695	.873	1.083	1.356	1.782	2.179	2.681	3.055
13	.128	.259	.394	.538	.694	.870	1.079	1.350	1.771	2.160	2.650	3.012
14	.128	.258	.393	.537	.692	.868	1.076	1.345	1.761	2.145	2.624	2.977
15	.128	.258	.393	.536	.691	.866	1.074	1.341	1.753	2.131	2.602	2.947
16	.128	.258	.392	.535	.690	.865	1.071	1.337	1.746	2.120	2.583	2.921
17	.128	.257	.392	.534	.689	.863	1.069	1.333	1.740	2.110	2.567	2.898
18	.127	.257	.392	.534	.688	.862	1.067	1.330	1.734	2.101	2.552	2.878
19	.127	.257	.391	.533	.688	.861	1.066	1.328	1.729	2.093	2.539	2.861
20	.127	.257	.391	.533	.687	.860	1.064	1.325	1.725	2.086	2.528	2.845
21	.127	.257	.391	.532	.686	.859	1.063	1.323	1.721	2.080	2.518	2.831
22	.127	.256	.390	.532	.686	.858	1.061	1.321	1.717	2.074	2.508	2.819
23	.127	.256	.390	.532	.685	.858	1.060	1.319	1.714	2.069	2.500	2.807
24	.127	.256	.390	.531	.685	.857	1.059	1.318	1.711	2.064	2.492	2.797
25	.127	.256	.390	.531	.684	.856	1.058	1.316	1.708	2.060	2.485	2.787
26	.127	.256	.390	.531	.684	.856	1.058	1.315	1.706	2.056	2.479	2.779
27	.127	.256	.389	.531	.684	.855	1.057	1.314	1.703	2.052	2.473	2.771
28	.127	.256	.389	.530	.683	.855	1.056	1.313	1.701	2.048	2.467	2.763
29	.127	.256	.389	.530	.683	.854	1.055	1.311	1.699	2.045	2.462	2.756
30	.127	.256	.389	.530	.683	.854	1.055	1.310	1.697	2.042	2.457	2.750
∞	.12566	.25335	.38532	.52440	.67449	.84162	1.03643	1.28155	1.64485	1.95996	2.32634	2.57582

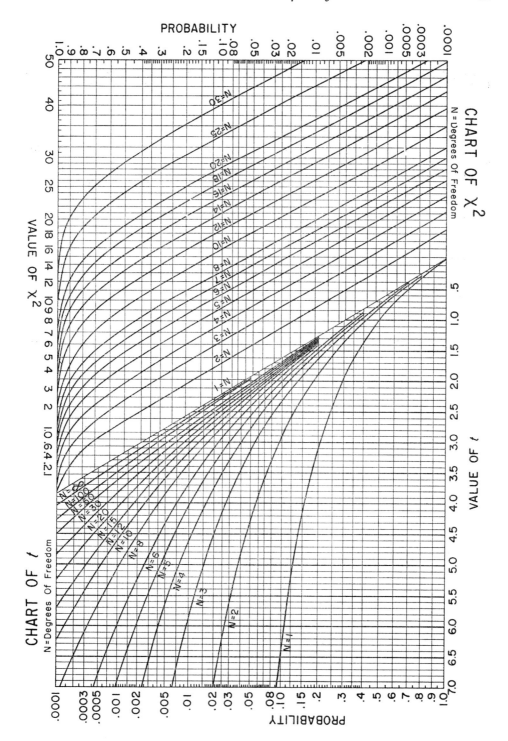

NUMBER OF PATIENTS NEEDED IN AN EXPERIMENTAL AND A CONTROL
GROUP FOR A GIVEN PROBABILITY OF OBTAINING A SIGNIFICANT RESULT
(ONE-SIDED TEST)

Smaller Proportion of Success (P_1)	Larger Minus Smaller Proportion of Success ($P_2 - P_1$)													
	.05	.10	.15	.20	.25	.30	.35	.40	.45	.50	.55	.60	.65	.70
.05	330	105	55	35	25	20	16	13	11	9	8	7	6	6
	460	145	76	48	34	26	21	17	15	13	11	9	8	7
	850	270	140	89	63	47	37	30	25	21	19	17	14	13
.10	540	155	76	47	32	23	19	15	13	11	9	8	7	6
	740	210	105	64	44	33	25	21	17	14	12	11	9	8
	1370	390	195	120	81	60	46	37	30	25	21	19	16	14
.15	710	200	94	56	38	27	21	17	14	12	10	8	7	6
	990	270	130	77	52	38	29	22	19	16	13	10	10	8
	1820	500	240	145	96	69	52	41	33	27	22	20	17	14
.20	860	230	110	63	42	30	22	18	15	12	10	8	7	6
	1190	320	150	88	58	41	31	24	20	16	14	11	10	8
	2190	590	280	160	105	76	57	44	35	28	23	20	17	14
.25	980	260	120	69	45	32	24	19	15	12	10	8	7	..
	1360	360	165	96	63	44	33	25	21	16	14	11	9	..
	2510	660	300	175	115	81	60	46	36	29	23	20	16	..
.30	1080	280	130	73	47	33	24	19	15	12	10	8	..	..
	1500	390	175	100	65	46	33	25	21	16	13	11	--	..
	2760	720	330	185	120	84	61	47	36	28	22	19	..	..
.35	1160	300	135	75	48	33	24	19	15	12	9	..	..	..
	1600	410	185	105	67	46	33	25	20	16	12	..	..	..
	2960	750	340	190	125	85	61	46	35	27	21	--	..	..
.40	1210	310	135	76	48	33	24	18	14	11	..	..	..	..
	1670	420	190	105	67	46	33	24	19	14	..	..	..	..
	3080	780	350	195	125	84	60	44	33	25	..	..	..	..
.45	1230	310	135	75	47	32	22	17	13	..	..	..	..	..
	1710	430	190	105	65	44	31	22	17	..	..	..	..	..
	3140	790	350	190	120	81	57	41	30	..	..	..	..	..
.50	1230	310	135	73	45	30	21	15	..	..	..	..	..	..
	1710	420	185	100	63	41	29	21	..	..	..	..	..	..
	3140	780	340	185	115	76	52	37	..	..	..	..	..	..

Upper Figure: Test of significance at .05 for α, power equals .8 for $(1-\beta)$.
Middle Figure: Test of significance at .05 for α, power equals .9 for $(1-\beta)$.
Lower Figure: Test of significance at .01 for α, power equals .95 for $(1-\beta)$.

NUMBER OF PATIENTS NEEDED IN AN EXPERIMENTAL AND A CONTROL
GROUP FOR A GIVEN PROBABILITY OF OBTAINING A SIGNIFICANT RESULT
(TWO-SIDED TEST)

Smaller Proportion of Success (P_1)	Larger Minus Smaller Proportion of Success (P_2-P_1)													
	.05	.10	.15	.20	.25	.30	.35	.40	.45	.50	.55	.60	.65	.70
.05	420	130	69	44	31	24	20	16	14	12	10	9	9	7
	570	175	93	59	42	32	25	21	18	15	13	11	10	9
	960	300	155	100	71	54	42	34	28	24	21	19	16	14
.10	680	195	96	59	41	30	23	19	16	13	11	10	9	7
	910	260	130	79	54	40	31	24	21	18	15	13	11	10
	1550	440	220	135	92	68	52	41	34	28	23	21	18	15
.15	910	250	120	71	48	34	26	21	17	14	12	10	9	8
	1220	330	160	95	64	46	35	27	22	19	16	13	11	10
	2060	560	270	160	110	78	59	47	37	31	25	21	19	16
.20	1090	290	135	80	53	38	28	22	18	15	13	10	9	7
	1460	390	185	105	71	51	38	29	23	20	16	14	11	10
	2470	660	310	180	120	86	64	50	40	32	26	21	19	15
.25	1250	330	150	88	57	40	30	23	19	15	13	10	9	..
	1680	440	200	115	77	54	40	31	24	20	16	13	11	..
	2840	740	340	200	130	92	68	52	41	32	26	21	18	..
.30	1380	360	160	93	60	42	31	23	19	15	12	10	..	..
	1840	480	220	125	80	56	41	31	24	20	16	13	..	..
	3120	810	370	210	135	95	69	53	41	32	25	21	..	..
.35	1470	380	170	96	61	42	31	23	18	14	11	..	..	..
	1970	500	225	130	82	57	41	31	23	19	15	..	..	..
	3340	850	380	215	140	96	69	52	40	31	23	..	..	..
.40	1530	390	175	97	61	42	30	22	17	13	..	..	..	..
	2050	520	230	130	82	56	40	29	22	18	..	..	..	..
	3480	880	390	220	140	95	68	50	37	28	..	..	..	..
.45	1560	390	175	96	60	40	28	21	16	..	..	..	..	..
	2100	520	230	130	80	54	38	27	21	..	..	..	..	..
	3550	890	390	215	135	92	64	47	34	..	..	..	..	..
.50	1560	390	170	93	57	38	26	19	..	..	..	..	..	..
	2100	520	225	125	77	51	35	24	..	..	..	..	..	..
	3550	880	380	210	130	86	59	41	..	..	..	..	..	..

Upper Figure: Test of significance at .05 for α, power equals .8 for $(1-\beta)$.
Middle Figure: Test of significance at .05 for α, power equals .9 for $(1-\beta)$.
Lower Figure: Test of significance at .01 for α, power equals .95 for $(1-\beta)$.

SAMPLE SIZE (n) REQUIRED FOR A PRELIMINARY TRIAL (PHASE IIA)
IN TERMS OF GIVEN LEVELS OF THERAPEUTIC EFFECTIVENESS
AND REJECTION ERROR (β)

Permissible Rejection Error (β)	Level of Therapeutic Effectiveness (Per Cent)									
	5	10	15	20	25	30	35	40	45	50
5 Per Cent	59	29	19	14	11	9	7	6	6	5
10 Per Cent	45	22	15	11	9	7	6	5	4	4

NUMBER OF PATIENTS REQUIRED FOR SPECIFIED
RELATIVE PRECISION *

Relative Precision	.10	.15	.20	.25	.30	.35	.40
No. of Patients (n) Required	100	45	25	16	12	9	7

$$* \text{ Relative Precision} = \frac{\text{Standard Error } (\hat{p})}{\hat{p}} = \sqrt{\frac{(1-\hat{p})}{n\hat{p}}}$$

MULTIPLIER TO BE USED IN DETERMINING SIZE OF SAMPLE FOR A
COMPARATIVE CLINICAL TRIAL WITH SIZE FIXED

Power (1-β)	Two-sided Test			One-sided Test		
	Level of Significance (α)			Level of Significance (α)		
	.01	.05	.10	.01	.05	.10
.80	11.7	7.9	6.2	10.0	6.2	4.5
.90	14.9	10.5	8.6	13.0	8.6	6.6
.95	17.8	13.0	10.8	15.8	10.8	8.6

$$\text{Sample size n} = \text{(multiplier from table)} \ \frac{\sigma_d^2}{\delta^2} \ \text{for paired samples} \qquad \text{(i)}$$

$$\text{Sample size n} = \text{(multiplier from table)} \ \frac{2\sigma_p^2}{\delta^2} \ \text{for independent samples} \qquad \text{(ii)}$$

SIGNIFICANCE LEVEL RELATED TO VALUE OF Z

Two-sided Test	.60	.50	.40	.30	.20	.10	.050	.02	.010
One-sided Test	.30	.25	.20	.15	.10	.05	.025	.01	:005
Value of Z	.52	.67	.84	1.04	1.28	1.64	1.96	2.33	2.58

RANDOM DIGITS

00 19	16 50	68 44	27 76	75 69	30 55	67 55	34 07	83 13	68 21
99 45	59 93	18 53	11 63	47 28	48 61	96 14	42 91	76 42	16 63
24 99	30 33	96 60	20 76	57 24	16 78	35 85	83 68	97 64	73 24
38 52	40 71	18 37	79 41	00 13	70 11	91 93	94 30	51 44	69 51
54 47	79 13	04 11	40 93	12 07	35 08	70 77	46 86	02 54	18 34
71 63	99 98	25 11	95 10	40 46	48 94	50 70	98 78	42 13	22 74
25 02	52 18	14 56	96 22	77 27	16 89	47 18	39 13	46 71	32 69
08 80	11 27	39 80	09 09	37 04	66 30	30 15	31 92	02 13	26 56
14 15	47 10	57 25	91 51	34 38	84 37	88 30	42 30	83 58	83 27
75 18	04 87	01 60	84 04	77 43	34 22	77 76	45 85	56 56	82 19
71 23	54 79	47 54	11 42	61 86	84 35	92 09	17 80	43 97	70 61
46 14	24 14	75 62	64 85	74 00	07 33	95 85	25 96	41 79	21 62
22 39	15 25	22 57	80 55	42 32	56 05	25 66	59 87	08 22	20 66
62 73	84 17	52 29	07 20	63 07	59 50	30 91	68 69	50 61	14 66
12 20	57 11	95 10	13 53	19 05	44 71	50 10	01 05	40 09	85 20
90 10	45 22	21 13	77 25	59 42	37 76	49 62	92 90	45 29	15 85
44 54	33 24	87 68	67 41	64 22	73 98	38 31	82 56	44 71	63 36
81 44	13 61	81 06	34 87	28 79	06 15	64 10	97 35	01 27	63 78
85 16	64 93	09 88	08 89	21 30	89 29	48 32	02 01	13 45	56 80
09 86	82 34	50 09	12 97	40 88	91 79	68 83	76 74	43 67	45 16
88 50	07 15	40 93	08 89	84 22	84 85	14 49	50 92	17 87	70 89
30 73	24 15	36 63	05 47	65 29	45 93	51 90	08 89	39 37	36 27
11 24	47 47	80 39	77 01	75 75	26 75	19 29	54 67	15 44	74 53
37 05	49 34	35 05	76 31	72 93	32 25	42 88	25 50	06 99	34 28
75 01	51 00	29 22	48 25	87 57	84 67	07 99	27 14	29 45	31 07
70 16	41 03	07 94	02 10	05 43	55 04	59 90	78 96	07 40	90 90
40 86	63 96	63 86	34 66	44 60	84 63	08 79	52 92	65 73	12 79
48 57	80 15	17 64	60 80	74 94	39 71	18 55	17 84	77 14	60 83
57 95	88 34	65 79	54 29	55 99	95 41	21 00	09 10	28 41	11 52
77 17	72 86	69 41	79 09	57 02	78 17	64 91	83 37	67 35	77 63
48 96	40 16	69 02	49 95	15 39	60 96	33 63	39 63	97 63	57 83
99 40	92 80	28 89	50 73	38 87	51 53	95 33	39 59	50 65	69 37
94 68	03 81	88 08	10 41	12 90	91 52	36 93	94 42	31 24	61 29
54 96	50 64	76 26	38 59	85 63	42 61	25 38	49 60	58 50	26 64
80 38	94 97	88 94	06 34	21 29	25 76	89 48	45 73	53 39	84 37
05 41	03 52	59 57	72 72	87 09	50 90	70 66	10 32	11 50	35 45
66 33	44 68	65 48	53 67	18 83	76 51	03 17	94 56	92 26	62 38
90 28	16 84	09 86	57 08	47 41	22 25	01 64	58 44	05 23	87 39
45 13	16 94	83 81	16 74	11 46	72 65	08 69	79 21	29 50	82 08
76 16	90 83	80 45	97 29	80 24	05 96	35 35	59 90	13 94	79 71
48 14	72 44	57 19	63 85	16 64	09 51	63 97	98 85	23 96	31 30
61 21	64 50	72 99	62 01	71 89	51 70	26 24	95 50	74 85	17 70
63 74	90 88	13 79	87 59	71 34	20 40	68 09	64 25	72 02	32 21
97 72	09 51	12 66	90 43	74 96	58 78	18 78	55 07	15 28	31 92
29 74	64 36	20 03	02 54	26 89	81 79	43 19	88 56	67 28	70 66
95 03	26 23	35 19	58 30	94 82	90 29	24 26	52 78	85 39	22 79
62 53	74 40	21 79	32 87	92 94	64 48	46 80	30 25	21 86	34 11
65 51	54 77	47 98	15 13	31 77	64 51	84 30	75 99	58 74	45 02
85 46	65 02	66 21	02 16	93 17	43 42	77 16	00 99	11 96	70 70
75 98	13 30	28 06	04 91	40 95	36 21	83 62	80 25	63 44	44 36

RANDOM DIGITS (Continued)

18 94	24 46	66 31	38 20	95 21	78 63	34 04	50 88	10 14	81 82
67 07	76 24	19 17	82 98	72 87	80 36	74 49	42 82	06 21	59 23
94 70	87 92	71 20	05 03	77 32	79 72	97 46	43 48	66 82	60 87
03 10	04 73	90 59	41 44	56 84	90 51	75 40	87 39	51 93	99 65
56 87	73 97	04 22	74 90	94 27	66 43	86 97	33 18	03 47	90 59
14 89	42 06	20 23	55 72	89 91	04 72	06 50	92 27	21 13	16 08
12 17	67 00	31 51	52 48	04 86	37 90	63 77	57 50	80 08	11 42
98 05	86 31	64 41	64 66	93 73	71 17	24 15	94 77	67 98	70 50
91 93	58 31	23 60	64 04	23 81	62 86	38 46	56 60	99 27	73 52
29 24	52 95	76 80	96 78	01 88	66 22	17 34	04 15	01 25	22 48
88 24	58 24	72 48	23 85	60 21	03 59	46 62	32 74	09 69	84 90
62 89	39 68	39 19	55 06	40 26	77 21	28 18	35 62	19 68	42 41
26 84	91 94	26 56	90 51	05 34	85 85	54 94	62 05	71 08	68 04
70 94	06 23	66 39	72 88	62 84	62 74	59 22	77 98	61 44	64 78
39 26	91 20	06 17	25 58	32 06	27 43	60 28	71 13	43 61	37 76
87 94	81 39	47 90	53 47	05 39	02 68	29 92	07 35	18 92	93 60
96 65	94 90	62 01	67 07	68 54	37 85	44 20	90 99	63 88	12 52
24 23	09 95	88 75	05 57	19 78	50 56	44 85	59 48	66 56	72 84
67 84	70 56	39 07	30 28	08 64	01 58	45 51	00 91	70 16	71 94
09 53	51 98	12 12	87 55	51 11	00 80	36 17	73 17	79 18	34 08
64 12	69 43	08 51	48 45	21 53	57 40	13 19	74 48	39 39	72 82
29 52	46 90	86 14	72 78	20 42	83 32	42 74	17 22	14 21	34 10
33 20	27 75	30 00	65 79	23 06	86 34	02 40	40 71	98 31	36 36
17 87	55 00	37 39	48 41	75 32	97 94	88 49	13 60	83 39	94 72
64 99	26 51	07 07	95 36	71 25	20 69	75 85	72 24	71 41	18 85
66 26	88 68	13 67	60 43	71 05	01 07	22 52	69 09	67 55	57 60
71 46	22 44	97 87	54 23	48 62	86 68	73 19	13 60	28 00	78 55
14 85	46 13	58 46	17 15	44 61	57 77	83 42	28 07	36 69	66 28
03 33	62 42	43 97	88 59	93 69	93 12	10 90	61 70	91 09	51 13
85 72	59 79	59 61	63 93	44 28	69 77	50 27	58 93	38 17	88 11
65 93	94 15	79 53	01 07	44 13	78 80	75 06	11 18	70 42	46 18
21 81	72 19	34 69	41 39	77 10	95 24	42 89	86 48	15 28	88 52
96 81	85 29	83 55	93 06	54 27	30 85	69 68	77 11	82 27	77 37
93 78	51 64	15 68	39 79	36 91	69 42	33 81	83 06	18 83	70 13
67 50	63 79	37 53	34 19	49 19	86 73	82 95	07 57	18 40	38 63
37 40	60 23	95 27	61 92	75 23	40 71	34 45	30 72	74 19	89 22
72 07	91 71	51 07	71 87	78 12	32 37	33 96	98 53	26 81	39 01
83 82	86 69	97 40	07 17	77 72	34 04	18 01	66 88	66 31	61 99
64 86	85 24	18 00	92 95	29 52	08 84	62 39	23 56	66 64	08 55
45 40	56 60	34 59	89 16	08 56	53 97	41 62	26 29	05 16	73 26
09 95	93 23	65 45	50 40	70 39	40 10	23 72	90 96	99 85	87 81
19 45	32 44	14 38	99 44	85 29	40 29	30 14	91 38	34 22	99 90
04 86	46 88	58 40	67 24	72 30	94 43	52 29	40 62	82 07	13 43
72 47	15 98	57 56	29 80	46 63	88 32	84 22	63 83	44 37	61 69
40 91	92 97	22 16	30 34	86 60	91 87	54 99	93 36	15 18	12 37
67 35	65 53	90 61	65 71	75 79	46 63	75 12	69 72	55 81	12 00
62 84	23 20	45 37	86 56	31 43	70 30	97 77	64 98	24 14	17 14
96 03	40 48	74 86	63 31	41 73	04 61	88 65	10 69	30 34	80 78
90 22	12 15	25 97	53 75	52 89	22 58	47 68	57 75	20 50	14 73
80 13	85 78	34 82	22 48	20 84	82 35	80 90	73 82	76 77	82 46

AUTHOR INDEX

SUBJECT INDEX

A

Acceptance or rejection of hypothesis, 9, 32
Adjustment for differences
  in one factor in cases and controls, 17, 18,
    61-64
  in one subclassification, 50
Adjuvant therapy and mammary carcinoma,
    39, 58
Age adjustment, 6
Aims
  of comparative clinical trial, 28
  of retrospective studies, 10
Alternative hypothesis (and test), 9, 13, 41,
    50, 69, 71
American Medical Association, 85
Analysis
  comparison of average values, 40-42, 68-71
  comparison of percentages, 39, 40, 58-64
  end-points for, 6
  of survival time, 42-46, 72-78
  principles of, 9, 39
  see also Prospective studies, Retrospective
    studies
Antagonism between tuberculosis and cancer,
    19
Anticoagulants, comparison of, 28, 29
Antimalarial action, cinchona and, 3
Arrangement of data
  for chi-square test, 58
  from matched samples, relative risk, 66
  to test a difference in proportions, 62
Association
  between characteristic and disease, 10, 21
  causal significance of statistical, 21
  chi-square test of, 13, 14, 50, 58-61
  consistency of, 11
  dose response and, 11
  false, between disease and characteristic(s),
    19
  or difference in proportions, 58, 61
  specificity of, 11
  strength of, 11, 22
Autopsies, consecutive, as control group, 19
Average values, 51, 52
  arithmetic mean, 51
  comparison of two
    in paired data, 40, 68, 69
    in unpaired data, 41, 69-71

median, 52
size of sample for, 37, 38
standard error of, 53

B

Bayesian trials, 31
Berkson-Gage method, 44
Bias
  in clinical trials, 28, 29
  in retrospective studies, 11, 12, 19, 20
  in studies of matched samples, 15
Brain Tumor Study Group, 43
Bronchogenic carcinoma, 9, 11, 12, 17-19, 21,
    64, 65

C

Calculations, *see* Appendices
Carcinoma
  bronchogenic, 9, 11, 12, 17-19, 21, 64, 65
  mammary, 39, 58
  of the colon, 30
  of urinary bladder, 10
  see also Smoking
Cases and controls, 11
  adjustment for differences in one factor, 17,
    66
  measures of relative risk in, 65
  retrospective study of, 12, 19
Categories of patients for sudy, 30
Causal
  criteria, 6, 11
  inference, 17, 21, 22
  relationship to dose response, 22
Censored observations, 41-43, 72
Chance of
  false-negative statement, 32
  false-positive statement, 32
Chart of chi-square and t, 55, 91
Chi-square tests
  adjusting for differences in one factor,
    61-64
  chart for, 55
  definition of, 50
  for independent samples, 58-60
  for matched samples, 16, 17, 60, 61
  of association, 13, 14, 50, 58-61
  of relative risk, 65-67

[99]